A
STUTTERING
REVOLUTION

Don't fix your stutter, fix your life

Paul Gaskin

First published in Great Britain by Practical Inspiration Publishing, 2024

ISBN   9781788604895   (print)
       9781788604918   (epub)
       9781788604901   (mobi)

Want to bulk-buy copies of this book for your team and colleagues? We can customize the content and co-brand *A Stuttering Revolution* to suit your business's needs.

Please email info@practicalinspiration.com for more details.

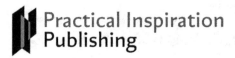

To the millions of people around the world who stutter.
It's time to live the life you really want.

Table of contents

Acknowledgements

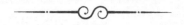

I would like to thank a wide range of people who have supported me in writing and publishing the book after a very long gestation period.

My first thanks must go to my soulmate and wife Christine who lit up my life when I met her at 15 years of age, and who has always been confused as to why I stutter. To her I was just Paul. My brilliant kids Victoria and Jonathan who are better people than I will ever be and have been hugely supportive of me writing the book.

A big thank you to Alan Robertson, who has been a friend and mentor for nearly 30 years. It was Alan who first said over 20 years ago 'I think you have a book in you Gaskin'. He has kept pushing and encouraging me until it was done.

The biggest thank you has to go to Alison Jones and her team at Practical Inspiration Publishing. What a team. They have dragged me kicking and screaming to produce a better book than I ever imagined. A notable mention to Alison Gray, who gave me clarity and detail to structure the book in a much clearer way.

There have been a number of people who have given their time and constructive feedback to the evolution of the book including David Fox, Oliver Blackwell, Chris Welford and John Russell.

Bob McGuiness, a former Divisional Serco CEO, played a significant part in my career and gave me the space and support to be the leader I became. A man of high integrity, who has also supported the writing of the book and who is featured in the story at the end of the book.

Going back over my career there are people I want to mention who have played a pivotal role in helping me become who I am today. I had some brilliant teachers. I am sorry I can't remember you all but a few stand out. Des Seabrook needs a double mention, teacher, rugby coach and a character of immense depth, humility and talent. Rob Brewer, who gave me the step up I needed in my higher education. Andrew Walsh, Liz Weatherhogg, Bernie Waldron, Terry Standing, Norman Wallwork, Maurice Hesford, John Lomax, Ian Grant from BAE Systems. People in work who shaped the early part of my career and allowed me to fail, succeed and develop. Phil Vernon, David Koch and Stephen Bayliffe from PricewaterhouseCoopers. George Miles, Nick Brown, David Campbell and Kevin Craven from Serco. And a whole range of colleagues too numerous to mention but you know who you are and the bonds we all formed through many difficult and challenging times.

A notable mention to Francis White, Clare Sadler and Rebecca Jeffs who have given me great support and challenge throughout parts of my career – offering a supporting hand when I was deep down a well looking for a rope. A big thank you to Steven Halliday and Kirsten Howells at STAMMA, who have been hugely supportive and inspirational in making life better for people who stutter.

I want to thank the strangers who have encouraged me after a terrible presentation, when I have felt as though I have let the side down, sick, ashamed and embarrassed. Sometimes people just appear and say words of encouragement without explanation of who they are or why they are saying encouraging words. To all those people a heartfelt thank you.

Lastly my mum and dad who forged me into what they could and then stood back and tried to help. But I think I was always on a different track. I knew I wanted more, I knew I could do more. And after all these years that fire is still burning away. I am not finished yet.

Introduction

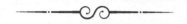

Don't be defined by your stutter

Joe Biden, the president of the United States, has publicly stated that his mother would say his stutter didn't define him – essentially reminding him that he was more than his stutter. She was absolutely right.[1] He is, and became, so much more. So can you!

You don't need fixing!

For most of my life people (parents, teachers, doctors, speech therapists, friends, work colleagues and even random strangers) have told me that I was broken and I should get that fixed. But I wasn't broken. I was OK. I just stuttered.

I want you to believe and trust that you are not broken. You don't need to be fixed. I want 'a stuttering revolution'. I want you to focus on what you really want to become. What you are good at. What you love to do and how to achieve a rich and fulfilling life. The life you really want. Not a life you or others believe has been restricted by your stutter.

I know your stutter can be all-consuming. So much so that it dominates every aspect of your life. You can start to believe that you are limited. And most of the help, support and advice available is to help improve the way you speak.

---

[1] Shahbaz, 'What Joe Biden's speech disorder means for young Americans with disabilities', 2020.

What if there is a different way? What if the 70 million adults around the world who are estimated to stutter were given the tools to believe they could be whatever they wanted to be, by focusing on what is great about them? What if we helped people like you to decide what you really want from your life, to find a job you love, to discover what you are already good at and to develop a superpower? How empowering would that be? I want a revolution in thinking. You can be whatever you want to be in life despite having a stutter. Your stutter is a part of you. It's not all of you.

Searching for a cure

My parents spent many years trying everything the UK National Health Service and private medicine had to offer to find out what was wrong with their son – looking for a cure to fix him and his speech. I love them for that. It must have been very difficult and a worry. If only they could have known I was going to be OK.

Stop!

At 17, I made a decision to stop all medical treatments to help me with my speech. It would be what it would be. I would take on life and not let my stutter stop me from being who I wanted to be. Even after that decision, I have spent a lifetime struggling to breathe, trying to overcome blocks, and paralysis in my neck, throat and face. Sometimes, my stutter was so bad, it felt like my face would get stuck trying to speak. I had days when I felt shame, humiliation, despair, upset and absolute frustration. I had days when I didn't want to live. It got that bad. It's hard to explain how exhausting daily life can be. The battle with the voices in your head. The anticipation, planning, rehearsal, stuttering, physical reaction, reflection, self-analysis, self-criticism, chastisement. Just to speak or, worse, say my name.

No excuses

I have days, even today, when I find it a real struggle to speak. I can still have huge ups and downs. These days are few in number. I now have the perspective to say to myself, I'm having a bad day. I stutter. So what! And move on. I have learned that my demons (the voices in my head) go beyond my stutter. I have therefore spent my lifetime trying to be a better me, stutter and all. I have learned I can't use my stutter as an excuse for any failures, lack of success or for not having the courage to become a better version of me.

Inspiration for this book

In this book I share stories from early childhood, high school, starting work and throughout my career to describe how I dealt, or at times didn't deal very well, with life. I describe the decisions I made to make my stutter less important to who I was and the person I wanted to become. I hope you find the stories relatable to your own experiences. From an early age, I decided not to take myself too seriously. That's how I got through many shitty situations and to have a really enjoyable and rewarding life. I wouldn't swap my life with anyone else's. I have become more than I ever thought I would be. I want to help you believe you can be so much more.

I have included a list of acknowledgements to thank all the brilliant people who have helped me on my journey to write and publish the book as well as people from life who I owe a great deal to.

Experience can give you wisdom

I also want to share some of my realizations with you. As the old adage goes, if I knew then what I know now, my life would be very different. I knew I wanted to become more than my stutter. I wanted more in my life. And more out of me. But I didn't know what that really meant. Or where to start. I have therefore tried over 20 jobs to find one I loved. I have tried hundreds of self-help tools to achieve more in my life. I have failed a lot. But through failure and mistakes I have learned a great deal about what does and doesn't work in my personal and work life. I will share all of this with you.

Through my own life journey, I have realized that life is hard. At times, it is likely to be a struggle. I thought the struggling was just me, because I had a stutter. Nope! Here is the learning. Everyone has life struggles and demons to overcome. Everyone has things that go wrong and competing voices in their heads. Your progress and real growth will be achieved by you overcoming and working through your struggle. This will be a lifelong process. Not a one-time event! But as someone smarter than me once said, 'Would you rather struggle to achieve something you love or struggle with a life you don't much care for?' As you will read later in the book, 80% of people are in jobs they don't like. They're struggling for what?

To quote Bruce Willis, 'I learned so much from having to deal with stuttering. It gave me insight into other people's pain, other people's suffering. It made me understand that everyone has something they're fighting to overcome and sometimes trying to hide.'[2]

What do you want from your life?

The first step is to make a decision. Sure, you have a stutter. But decide you want more from your life and that your stutter will not hold you back from what you want to become! You may want to become famous, to improve your life a little, to get the job you really want, to say what you feel to your partner, to earn a bit more money, or to feel less shy when meeting new people. Whatever your ambition, big or small, this book will help you. Darren Sproles, former American football star said,

---

[2] Lee, 'Bruce Willis gets emotional in speech on stuttering', 2016.

'I remember a long time ago, my grandpa told me, "Don't let anybody tell you, you can't do anything, because you stutter."'[3]

A five-step process to become so much more than your stutter

From my own experiences and years of learning, I have designed a simple five-step process to help you achieve what you want from your life, to help you be the person you want to be, to feel proud of who you are and to feel better about yourself than you do today. I want you to know that by focusing on what you are good at and turning that strength into a superpower, you will quickly start to make changes to how you think and feel and ultimately what you do.

Each step uses tools and techniques that I have used and have proven to work in my personal life and throughout my 40-year career. I have incorporated thinking from the world's best self-help experts, including David Goggins, Tony Robbins, Joe Dispenza, Vikesh Lukhiani, Tom Bilyeu, Mel Robbins, Stephen R. Covey, Jordan B. Peterson and so many more. I have drawn inspiration from famous people who stutter (or have stuttered), including Ed Sheeran, Samuel L. Jackson, Tiger Woods, Emily Blunt, Darren Sproles, Julia Roberts, Joe Biden, Bruce Willis, Winston Churchill and others who have motivated me through their stories of despair and hardship to succeed in life.

A friend to guide you

If I have missed anyone out of the book or got some of the details slightly wrong, it is not with the intent of any offence. I am just trying to tell a simple story of a boy who struggled to make sense of the world with a stutter and to say his name. I know there are many people with

---

[3] Stuttering Foundation, 'Darren Sproles', 2021.

a stutter who have achieved so much more than me. They can be your beacon and inspiration of what you can ultimately achieve. If that's what you want. This book will provide you with a step-by-step and practical process to achieve whatever you want. A bit more. A lot more. Or just to be happier with yourself.

Above all I want this book to be practical. I have provided a series of exercises that will guide you to decide what you want from your life, to learn the skills and to find the people you need to meet to achieve your goals.

Lazaro Arbus, a Cuban-born pop singer with a stutter, said, 'The things that normal people think are so easy become so hard for me.' So maybe if you work through this book your life will become a bit easier.[4]

I spent many years thinking I was alone. That I had to be fixed. And someone would come along with a cure and save me. You are not alone. You are not broken. This is your little book of hope, companionship and practical help. So what are you waiting for?

Two stories to illustrate my journey

I want to share two stories that show the progress I made from feeling like a victim and being dominated by my stutter to knowing my stutter was now a part of me and not all of me. The first story describes a humiliating event at work, when I was 17 years of age, in front of over 100 people, in an apprentice training school in Bolton in Lancashire. The second was a defining moment, when I spoke as a senior leader to an audience of 1,200 people, from over 30 countries around the world, before the launch of the iconic Dubai Metro, the first urban train network in the Middle East.

---

[4] Hill, 'Stuttering "American Idol" contestant steals the spotlight', 2022.

In my first job, I wore the wrong boots

I was 17 and having a number of treatments for my stutter, including speech therapy and hypnotherapy. I had started work as an apprentice missile technician at BAE Systems, as my dad didn't think I was bright enough to do A-level exams (advanced exams you take in the UK when you are age 16–18, prior to university). I earned GBP 25 per week. I left home at 5:30 a.m. every day to catch two buses to get to work on time. I really didn't know what the hell I was doing or where I was going. My speech was at its worst. I had days when I couldn't speak. My anxiety and feelings of not being good enough were also playing hugely in my life.

My first year of training was shared with 100 mechanical and 20 electronic apprentices. The training school was located underground and next to a farm. It was not the best environment. Some days, pigs escaped from the farm and ran riot through the training school. The machine shop smelled of coolant (a fluid used to cool the hot metal on the machines). In summer, it was unbearably hot, dirty and smelly. In my first week, I was caught wearing steel-capped training shoes, a gift from my dad who had worked in factories all his life (training shoes were a complete no-no in a machine shop). My dad thought steel-capped training shoes would be something no one else would have. He was right!

A stuttering fail

'You with the training shoes on!' shouted one of the instructors.

Over 100 apprentices stared directly at me, as the instructor shouted down the long, narrow corridor of the training school, where we all were about to sit to have our morning coffee break.

'What's your name?'

Oh shit! Not that question. My face and neck immediately turned red. I clenched my fist, turned around to face the instructor who was marching down to confront me. And the nightmare started. A little bead of sweat now sat on my eyebrow. My neck was tense. And the voices in my head burst into life.

'P-P-P-P-P-P-P-P... ... ... P-P-P-P-P-P-P... ... ... P-P-P-P-P-P-P-P... P-P-P-P-P-P-P-P-P,' I said. My tongue pressed so hard against my teeth it made them hurt. My throat started that infernal clicking sound. *Could anyone hear that? They are all looking at me. Shit. Shit.* I was getting hotter and hotter. 'P-P-P-P-P-P... P-P-P-P-P-P-P-P-P-P-P-P-P-P-P-P-P-P,' I said, valiantly trying to force out my damn name.

Sometimes, when I stutter, it can feel like the world completely slows down. My face is contorted. The voices in my head are frantically looking for a way out of the situation. Yet, part of my brain is able to look and observe what is going on around me in great detail. It's what I imagine an out-of-body experience is like. The voice trapped behind my teeth. But my eyes and ears are super sensitized. This doesn't work if my eyes become tight shut, which sometimes happens. Two parts of a scene in a film. Part one of the film is in my head. I'm not going to lie. It's all pretty shit! Part two is what everyone can see.

'Stop!' the instructor shouted, 'You – supervisor's office now!'

I put my head down. I looked at my bloody steel-capped training shoes and walked to the gallows. As I passed the sitting apprentices, I knew my nickname was going to become the 'Stuttering Scouser' (the Scouser reference will become clear in the next section). I was right. It was! I was a clairvoyant as well.

Inspiring a new workforce

Six months before the opening of the iconic Dubai Metro in March 2009, I stood on stage with the chief executive officer of Serco Integrated Transport, Nick Brown, and the managing director of Serco Middle East, Zafar Raja, looking out on a sea of 1,200 faces from over 30 countries around the world. We were in the process of hiring and training 2,000 people to launch the Dubai Metro at 9 minutes past 9:00 p.m.

on 9 September 2009. It was to be the longest driverless system in the world at the time and the first metro system in the Middle East. The launch was politically and economically significant to Dubai, as we were in the middle of a global financial crisis. A successful opening would signify to the world that Dubai was still open for business.

What stutter?

After Nick and Zafar gave their speeches and the applause died down, I looked out at the sea of expectant faces as they waited for me to speak. I was another stranger speaking to them about the next stage of their life in a foreign country. I sensed the feeling in the audience. I felt an immediate connection. I felt I knew exactly the right thing to say. This moment was about them. It was their story. I shared that I knew why they were here in Dubai: 99% of them had left their country of origin, their families and loved ones to earn and send money back home. I also spoke about their pride in making history in launching an iconic metro system. I'm told the speech really caught the moment and moved many to tears. At 17, I had days when I could barely speak; that day I was applauded for the way I spoke.

The culmination of a long struggle

On the evening of the launch, I was in the Metro control room which was far from finished. There were wires, equipment and people everywhere. Sheikh Mohammed bin Rashid Al Maktoum, vice president and prime minister of the UAE and ruler of Dubai, opened the Dubai Metro on the expected date and on time. He rode the Metro for two stops, and it was officially open. I was awarded the Serco Global Leadership Award for my role in the mobilization. The project was a huge success for Serco and our Metro team. They had overcome what many had believed to be unassailable obstacles to open on time. I had learned a lot and was hugely proud of the team.

I became more than my stutter

I went on to hold many senior roles in Serco. I lived and worked in India, Hong Kong and Dubai before returning to the UK. My final job, before leaving Serco in 2021, was UK and Europe human resources director. I worked with the chief executive officer (CEO) and the executive management team to run a GBP 2 billion per year division comprising six business units, across 10 countries and employing approximately 38,000 people. I was one of four divisional HR directors on the global HR leadership team reporting to the chief operating officer (COO) of a GBP 5 billion per year organization employing 60,000 people globally. All well beyond anything I could have imagined as a 17-year-old apprentice earning GBP 25 per week and travelling to work on two buses. The question is how?

Your story

You have your story. Where you started. Where you are now and where you are going. I can offer you my real-life experiences and help from the people I have learned the most from to make my life better. For a moment I want you to imagine that you cannot fail. Liberate your mind to dream and think big about your future. What if you could achieve anything or be the person you really want to be? What if? What springs to mind? You may just want a bit more than you have today. It doesn't matter. You have chosen to become more. Whatever that means for you.

How to get the most from the book

The book is divided into three main parts followed by the appendices and a reference list.

Part 1: My life and lessons learned

I share stories from my childhood and starting work. I describe my life with a stutter and finding a book that changed my life. Hopefully you will find many of my experiences relatable to yours. I will ask you questions about your stutter and the impact it had on you and those around you as you grew up. I suggest that you read all of Part 1 before starting Part 2. You might go back to Part 1 in the future to remind yourself of a story that might help you in everyday life or a quote that you found useful. However, the main focus of the book is Part 2: Your life, using the lessons learned!

Part 2: Your life, using the lessons learned

This part is your five-step self-help manual. The aim of the self-help manual is to help, guide and support you to become more than your stutter and to focus on what is great about you. Each of the five steps poses a question at the start of the section, which you are then helped to answer using a series of exercises.

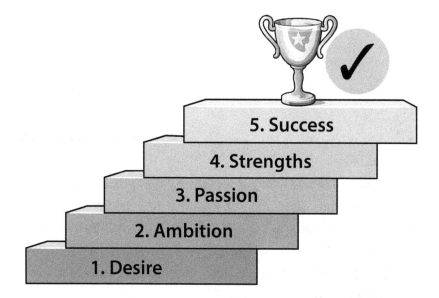

Fig. 1 Five steps to create, live and love the life you really want.

The five steps

Step 1: Desire – How determined are you to become more than your stutter?

Step 2: Ambition – What do you really want from your life?

Step 3: Passion – How will you find the job you love, and love the job you do?

Step 4: Strengths – What are you already really good at? What is your superpower?

Step 5: Success – How will you get what you want?

I recommend that you read Part 2 a step at a time. Each of the five steps has a number of exercises that will take you some time to work through to get the most out of them. As you complete each step, you will fill in your **Success Summary Sheet** (see Appendices). You will use the Success Summary Sheet to capture the outputs from each of the five steps on a single page. This single page will be incredibly useful as a daily reference document and reminder of your goals, actions and key learning points from the five steps. You may want to share what you're learning about yourself along the way with a trusted partner or friend. It often helps to makes sense and consolidate your learning by chatting it through with someone else.

In Step 5, we're going to learn five new skills to deliver your life goals:

- Skill 1: Success Action Process – translating your thoughts into actions
- Skill 2: Mental Metal – developing your mental strength
- Skill 3: Time-shifting – making time to create your new life
- Skill 4: Success Workbook – reflecting on what does and doesn't work
- Skill 5: Brilliant Networking – finding role models to get you faster results

Part 3: Conclusion

I pull the key themes of the book together and share my rationale for why I believe we need 'a stuttering revolution'. I also share a very personal story about a moment in my life when I had a thought that changed my life. A life-changing thought about my stutter. It's a revelation that caused me to focus on don't fix your stutter, fix your life! I'm hoping it will give you an insight and the confidence to change the way you see yourself and live your life.

Appendices

Success Summary Sheet
Organizations with contact details – support for people who stutter
Further resources

In researching this book, I have been blown away by the advancement and support for people who stutter. Whether it's the research that has been undertaken by the medical profession, the range and sophistication of speech therapies, the stunning work of the stuttering bodies including STAMMA (The British Stuttering Association), The American Stuttering Association, The Michael Palin Centre or the many training and support programmes that are now available. All dedicating their intelligence, energy and passion to help people who stutter improve their ability to communicate. I have included contact details for a number of organizations you could find helpful.

I'm hoping that *A Stuttering Revolution* offers a complementary approach that works in conjunction with the current support available. But moreover, that it offers more accessible help and guidance to a wider range of people.

Further resources

I have provided links to resources that can help people who have read the book.

Together we all have the same aim. We are all people and organizations trying to help people who just happen to speak differently. That's because we all know that people who stutter have something valuable to offer the world. And the world will be a better place if we have the confidence to do so.

Please share the material with other people; it applies equally to people who don't stutter. How can that be, I hear you say? Because we're all people. We just happen to speak differently.

Your Success Workbook

Your Success Workbook is a journal or a note pad. It's a place to capture your thoughts and answers to the exercises and questions, as you progress through the book. It will become your companion, your reference document and a place to capture your learning along the way. I would invest in a decent note pad, as it's going to be used to create and design your new life and capture all the new and powerful things you will be learning about yourself.

My hope for you

I want this book to help you to change your mind about your life with a stutter and ultimately for you to change your life. Since my early 20s, I have read hundreds of books to help me become a better me. Every book I have read has given me at least one nugget or piece of learning that I have used to shape my life.

There are some books that stand out as helping me with my life, and have given me aha! moments. This is a list of a few of the many from which I have drawn on in this book: *The 7 Habits of Highly Effective People*, Stephen R. Covey; *How to Win Friends and Influence*

People, Dale Carnegie; *Awaken the Giant Within*, Tony Robbins; *Feel The Fear and Do it Anyway*, Susan Jeffers; *The Seven Spiritual Laws of Success*, Deepak Chopra; *The Monk Who Sold His Ferrari*, Robin S. Sharma; *Words That Change Minds*, Shelle Rose Charvet; *True North*, Bill George; *First, Break All the Rules*, Marcus Buckingham and Curt Coffman; *P.H.D.12 The Elements of Great Managing*, Rodd Wagner and James J. Harter and so many more.

But the first book I read that caused an interrupt and really changed my life was *The 4%* by Dr Gerald Kushel. I hope in some small way that *A Stuttering Revolution* helps you have your aha! moments.

Good luck!

Part 1

My life and lessons learned

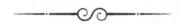

Early years

In this section, I share stories from my early childhood, the shock of my challenging birth for my mum, the shock I had finding out I had a stutter, the start of my parents' journey looking for a cure to fix their son and the emergence of the voices in my head.

A Scouser is born

I was born breech in labour lasting a very long time in Broadgreen Hospital, Liverpool at 7:42 a.m. on Friday, 2 November 1962. I have often wondered if that breach delivery caused my life of struggle. A struggle to breathe. A struggle to speak. A struggle to be better. A struggle to make my life mean something. But mainly a struggle just to say what I wanted to say. My name!

People born in Liverpool are called Scousers. We are passionately proud of it. There is a bite to our humour. A tough attitude to life. An enduring ability to be self-deprecating. And to fearlessly keep ourselves and others grounded. I'm called a plastic Scouser, as I moved away from Liverpool at the age of three. I don't have a strong accent, just a twang. However, if I ever hear 'You'll Never Walk Alone' (the famous Liverpool Football Club anthem) it always makes me stand up taller and puff out my chest, and brings an uncontrollable tear to my eye. I associate myself with the city that has had to fight to survive and be heard. I'm an avid Liverpool football supporter who finds it difficult to watch a game without feeling sick. I hate to lose and Liverpool losing is the worst.

My mum, Miriam (always known to my dad as Marion) and my dad, Ernest Alan (known as Alan) Gaskin came from humble beginnings. My dad was a toolmaker who worked shifts in car factories all his life. My mum started work on the Plessey Electronics production line in Kirby before finding her passion for nursing, which she did for 33 years at Billinge Hospital near Wigan before it was demolished.

My story began in a small house in Merton Grove, Childwall, in Liverpool. I was the first child. We had a dog named Jip. My dad had a motorbike and sidecar and I had a sandpit in the garden. My mum tells a story that when I was nearly three years of age, I woke up one night, got out my trike and rode naked at 3 a.m. to find the park at the end of the road. Luckily, I was spotted and brought home by a neighbour coming home from a late shift. From what I remember, life as a very young child was good. Hornby® train sets, pedal cars and playing with kids on our road.

When I was three, we moved to a two-bedroom bungalow in Billinge near Wigan, Lancashire, midway between Liverpool and Manchester. The move from Liverpool to a rural village caused huge issues for my mum, who was already seen as the black sheep of her family. My mum's relationship with her mum, and a perceived lack of love, would cause many issues for me as a child. In 1965, my brother David was born and our little family was complete.

I attended the St James Infant and Primary School in Billinge, which was within a quarter of a mile of the St James Catholic Infant and Primary School my future wife attended, unbeknown to me, one school year ahead of me.

I still remember my first day at school, lining up in the school playground, having our names read out and being taken into the cloak room to hang up our coats and going into the classroom. We were given little blackboards and chalk to write our names. It all seemed so big and daunting. I still remember the smell of school meals, the dinner ladies (who always seemed old and had coloured hair tied in buns) with a swarm of clingy children around them. I wasn't one of them.

Billy the barber

Before starting school, my dad took me to Billy's Barbers in Lower Billinge. Billy would say, 'You can have any hairstyle you want, as long it's a number between a number 1 and 4.' My number, as stipulated by my dad, was always a 1, which resulted in shearing off all the hair from my head, giving me my first nickname at school. Hedgehog. It was great with the girls who would like to feel the little spikes on my head. Not so good with boys, who all thought I looked mean and wanted to fight. At that young age I was always in trouble with teachers. I had a desire to speak up, to be funny and to make people laugh. My dad had drilled into me to stick up for myself (a Scouse badge of pride). Don't let anyone push you around, not even the teachers. At a young age that can be unsophisticated advice. No matter how well intentioned.

As a result, I spent many a time sitting outside the office of Mr Alker, the headmaster of the infant and primary school, who always, like the dinner ladies, seemed very old. Only he smelled of tobacco from a pipe he constantly smoked and played with. Mr Alker would mentally scar me with a statement in my final year of primary school, 'Nothing good will ever come of you, Gaskin, mark my words.' His words haunted me until my early 30s.

I remember many of my early days of school with great fondness. I walked a mile and a half to and from school every day. Played football. Drew pictures. Made homemade bread. Wrote stories and chatted to friends. Life felt good, with a few little hiccups along the way.

I've got a what?

'Everything you think is wrong with you is actually right because that makes you an individual, and that makes you an even more interesting human. That makes you, you.'[5] Ed Sheeran talking about his stutter. If only I had known that back then.

In those early years of school, I was oblivious to any problem I had with my speech. I genuinely cannot remember it being an issue. However, it must have been a great concern to my parents. My mum used to say to people, 'they made our Paul change hands at school; he was left-handed, and they made him change to be right-handed, that's why he… gets, you know… stuck.' I didn't know what she meant, 'gets stuck'! But I do remember sometimes getting the looks of sympathy as though I was a sad little puppy with a broken leg. As I got older, I became increasingly aware of people either sniggering at me or adults trying to be helpful and saying things like 'take your time lad, and breathe'. I never felt like I was trying to rush. I was just trying to speak.

I do remember from those early days not being able to live up to the expectations of my dad. In any school report or activity, I never felt good enough. If I didn't get straight As or 100% in a test, he would chastise me and tell me I could do better. 'What do you mean three As and one B, what happened to the B?' he would ask. Today I understand what he was trying to do. His intention was to push me to be better. But that early imprinting into my memory of, I'm not good enough, would build a negative voice in my head that would cause me issues into adulthood.

David sings

The only other person I knew in my early childhood who had a stutter, because my mum told me, was David Maxwell, my brother's

---

[5] Stamurai, 'Do you know about Ed Sheeran's stuttering journey?', 2021.

best friend, who lived at the end of our road. When David Maxwell came to the door to ask for my brother (who was also called David), he would sing, 'Is David in, please? I would like to go out to play.' Poor lad, I thought, that's just weird. My mum asked me to sing sentences. I thought it sounded ridiculous. David didn't sound like himself. I felt it was more embarrassing than my stutter. I was having none of it!

Brains, my first role model

The call sign of *Thunderbirds*, the animatronic children's show, was FAB. I was never sure what it stood for, but I loved the programme. It had a futuristic theme, with space stations, clever flying machines with a pod in Thunderbird 2 that could deliver specialized equipment to the disaster area. I loved the character, Brains. He had a stutter. I'd never seen or heard anyone who spoke the way I did. He was also very clever. He was the smart guy behind the way the *Thunderbirds* team worked. I know it sounds very silly now, but the fact that I could see on the TV, someone (I know Brains was a puppet!) who was famous and had a stutter just made what I had a little less freaky (only a bit, ha!). It also starred Lady Penelope. She had a pink Rolls Royce and a butler called Parker. The *Thunderbirds* mission was to respond and help people who were in danger around the world. When an emergency happened, they would be transported from the control room on seats that went horizontal and took them underground to their Thunderbird. They then took off through a swimming pool or from inside a volcano. Brilliant.

Always top table

All through infant and primary school I sat on a table with the top five smartest kids in the class. Each class of 35 at school were graded into tables based on the teacher's view of our academic ability. At that time, in the final year of primary school, all pupils took a test called the eleven-plus. The eleven-plus was a set of tests that determined if you went to grammar or secondary modern school. I knew it was a big deal because the bright kids would go the grammar school and the 'thickies,' as they were called by school kids, would go to the secondary modern. I thought I would be all right. I was on the top table in my class and had been throughout the infant and primary school year. There was another class with pupils of the same age, that also had a top table, but I was told there would be enough places.

Will they put pipes down my throat?

My speech must have been getting worse because also in the last year of primary school, my parents decided to send me to see a psychologist and a speech therapist. I hadn't got a clue what that meant. I remember very clearly saying to my teacher, Mr Rochester, I was going to hospital to have tubes stuck down my throat to fix my stutter.

Mr Rochester said, 'I don't think so, it's more psychological.'

'More psychological,' I said with horror. 'What does that mean?'

He tapped his fingers on the side of his head.

Yikes, do I have something wrong inside my head? At that moment I was really confused. I didn't feel I had something wrong with me. My head felt great. I felt great. So what was it?

There's a voice in my head?

This conversation with Mr Rochester began the awakening of worry and the voices in my head. Up to that point, I don't really recall having a voice in my head. After that conversation, there it was, the voice of doubt. I now knew I had something wrong with me. I soon came to realize that the voice had many friends, all wanting space in my head. The voices seemed endless. The voice of rules, mainly: I can't do, don't do, shouldn't do, mustn't do, help others before yourself, be respectful, be strong, don't back down, you're not smart enough, it's not worth doing unless it's hard. S-o-o-o many negative voices. I did have good voices as well: have a go, you can do it, don't shuffle, hope, happy. It all just seemed so noisy. Where had they all come from?

What's a psychologist?

I went to see the psychologist. My mum and dad would go in first. Then I would be ushered in and asked lots of questions, such as how long had I stuttered? What did I think were the causes of the stutter? I didn't know I had a stutter. I didn't think it was a problem. It was just me.

The psychologist would ask: When does it get worse? I didn't know. Are there problems at home? I wasn't sure, as I didn't really know what that meant. All I remember from those meetings was that my mum used to do most of the talking. She always seemed upset. She would talk about her mum and her family. But I didn't understand that either. I then started speech therapy. That was the same process. The same sort of questions and then voice exercises, doing role play, making sounds on certain words. I met other kids who had stutters. But I never thought mine sounded like theirs, and some of them did seem anxious, but not me. I sometimes just couldn't say what I wanted to say.

As the sessions with the psychologist and the speech therapist continued, I started to feel anxious that I had something seriously wrong with me. I started to really worry what the hell it was. This made me very self-conscious, which seemed to make speaking worse, which in turn made me more self-conscious and so the spiral continued.

The label of the stutter and the fact that other people, including my parents, thought there was something wrong with me made the voices in my head start to grow and become even noisier. The voice in my head had become a choir.

Your story questions

- When did you know you had a stutter?
- What did people say caused it?
- How did it impact your life at the time?
- How were your parents and family?

A first life fail, at age 11

The eleven-plus results were in. The two classes who had taken the test (approx. 70 children) lined up in the school corridor. We walked up to Mr Alker's, the headmaster's office, in alphabetical order, to hear our pass or fail result. I remember walking up the wooden steps into Mr Alker's old and dark office. My feet made a loud noise on the wooden floor. It was a surreal moment. I seemed to notice lots of things in detail for the first time. The size of his desk with papers everywhere. Dust. So much dust. Cobwebs. The air musky. That dank, lingering tobacco smell. It all looked really old, but sharp in my mind. I clearly remember seeing his bald head with rather untidy grey bits of hair at the sides. Grey hairs coming out of his ears. The crinkles in his forehead and the little glasses perched on his nose, which he looked over when he spoke to you. There was a lot of noise and kids jostling outside the office door. Kids at that age can never keep still. His office seemed huge and time seemed to stand still as he looked up and said, 'Gaskin, failed'. It was terrible. My stomach felt like it dropped to my feet. I had failed my first big life test. 'Next,' he said, not looking at me. I stood there in shock.

Walk of shame

The walk of shame out of Mr Alker's office felt palpable. To this day, I can still remember the huge upset and embarrassment of walking past my friends, who had their thumbs up and down to understand where I was going. They all seemed as shocked as I was. But I was the one not going to grammar school. I was the one who had such a desperate sense of failure and loneliness.

My biggest worry was telling my dad. This would prove him right. This was a disaster. The feelings of failure were overwhelming. I just wanted to cry, and the pain in my chest, my stomach and my head made me feel as though I wanted to explode and run and run and run. But I had nowhere to go.

On my own

In the next few weeks, I went from being a happy, chatty chappie to the opposite. The embarrassment I felt was overwhelming. I had no one to talk to. What could I talk to my friends about? They were all getting excited about their new school. I felt they were no longer my friends, as we had nothing in common. I didn't want to go to my new school. I wasn't friends with anyone who would be going. I wondered if my failure was linked to my stutter. Was Mr Alker right? Would nothing ever good come of me? I felt I was going to the school for duffers, for practical and uneducated people. The negative voices in my head, the doubt, the worry, the apprehension was growing and becoming much louder.

The lows of high school

After the eleven-plus I was at a real low in terms of confidence. I went to high school (the secondary modern was renamed a high school) without any friends and feeling like a second-class citizen. In my first lesson, Mr Brown, the physical education teacher, got a cheeky and outspoken boy to the front of the class. He made him bend over and hit him with a huge sports pump. What a noise that made. Holy crap, I thought, I'm with the thickies and I'm going to get beaten. Thank goodness those were rare events. I later chatted with Mr Brown, who turned out to be a really nice guy and hugely supportive of me later on in my school life, as were most of the teachers.

I had decided that I wouldn't speak. I had failed my eleven-plus, I was at a new school with no friends and already being threatened by the big brother of someone I had fought with at primary school. I didn't want to draw attention to myself and my speech defect. I knew kids can be cruel. I could already hear that people were being given nicknames. I dreaded to think what mine would be. Break time was the worst. Kids would run out of class and head to the playground to chat in their groups. I had no one to hang out with. A school playground can be a big and lonely place if you're on your own.

Sam Neill, Irish-born actor and director, said: 'I was painfully shy because of it. When people said something to me I was afraid I'd have to reply, so I didn't say very much.'[6]

Silence is not golden

I remember making a decision about my stutter in an English class. I was 13 years of age. I would have a number of these moments in my life. But I know this was the first. It was a turning point. I sat in a class with 35 other children. The English teacher, Mr Hardman, led the conversation which revolved around characters in the book called *The Pearl*. After reading the book he asked, 'who was the stronger character, Kino or Jauna?'. Enthusiastic children stuck up their hands, wanting to speak and show how smart they were. The conversation flowed with lots of different opinions. The majority believed that Kino was the stronger character. I didn't agree. But I didn't speak. I had a point to make about Juana that no one else seemed to be making.

More people spoke. But no one made my point. I could see the clock on the wall ticking. Fifteen minutes to go before the end of class.

The voices in my head had an answer to the teacher's question, which I wanted to share, but I kept mum. Why didn't anyone see my point? I thought it was important. One voice in my head said, *maybe*

---

[6] Stuttering Foundation, 'Actor Sam Neill talks about stuttering', 2015.

you're just wrong; another voice, *you should say something; no, don't talk*, said another voice. Yet another voice said, *you can make your point about Juana. You can put your hand up and start the sentence with an 'I think'. 'I think' is OK for you. I's are easy to say, you know this, why are you waiting?'* Another voice said, *no, what if you stutter on the point? Worse what happens if you get a block? What happens if everyone laughs at you and you can't say Jauna?*

Tick-tock

The clock on the wall showed five minutes to go. *Go on put your hand up. Breathe in, breathe out. Jauna; it's too difficult to say, you can say something next week. Why don't you say, I think Jauna's… really quickly, c'mon I's are fine, breathe deeply and go! You might not get another chance? No one has mentioned Jauna. They're all missing the point. You can't say Jauna. What can you say instead? The lady in the book or woman in the book, Kino's wife; you can say Kino? Maybe not!* The voices were speeding up. *Just say the girl in the book, just say something for god's sake!* This conversation in my head is all happening very quickly and could often make me feel dizzy. The fighting between the voices was becoming incessant.

It's come out!

Then I blurted out, 'J-J-J-J-J-J-J-Jauana'.

Mr Hardman stopped and stared at me. Unimpressed. Hands on hips. 'Mr Gaskin, is it?' (Teachers often called you by your surname.) 'Hand not working? Can't be bothered to wait?'

The clock on the wall showed two minutes to go.

'What is your point, Mr Gaskin?'

The voice in my head said, *breathe. Shit, you've no breath left. Look at all the faces staring at you.* I blurted, 'I think that J-J-J-J-Jauna was the s-s-s-s-strongest of the t-t-t-t-t-two c-c-characters.' *Keep going.* My tongue was pushed against my teeth. My neck was choking, my eyes watering. And I made that god-awful clicking sound. *Can people hear that?* I blurted out, 'J-J-J-J-Jauna, f-f-f-f-f-f-followed her husband.' And then relief, the loud sound of the bell for the next class.

Better luck next time?

Walking out the door, I was red-faced. Out of breath. Exasperated and exhausted from the emotional and physical stress of wanting to speak.

Mr Hardman said, 'Mr Gaskin, it sounded like you started to make a point nobody else thought to make. Please speak up earlier next week and stick your hand up.'

Bless, Mr Hardman. All was not lost. He had unknowingly given me a little boost of confidence to ask a question next week.

More than that, in that moment, I decided regardless of what happened with my speech, I was going to speak. I had to speak. I was bursting with thoughts and ideas. I wanted to take part in the debate. I was going to say what I needed to say. Whatever the consequences and the fallout from other people's reactions. I had to push through. But I knew deep down it wasn't going to be easy. The embarrassment, the shame, the self-ridicule. Was I really sure I was ready? Or maybe now the problem (as people later in life tell me) was going to be shutting me up!

Your story questions

- What was life like for you at school?
- How did you cope?
- Were you singled out for being different?

In search of a cure

We can fix you

I don't know about you, but since I was a child people have been trying to fix me. My parents must have thought, surely it can't be that hard to fix a stutter? There must be a clever medical person, a tablet, a technique to stop that damn stutter? As any good parents would, my mum and dad turned to the medical professionals in the UK National Health Service (NHS) for help. I understand that the medical professionals are looking for a cause, a fault to be fixed. But no one ever assumed I was OK. I just had a stutter. Here's the conundrum. I never felt anxious until people kept asking me, why and when are you anxious? Why do you think you stutter? Are their times when you stutter more than others? Are you having problems at home? Then I learned to become anxious.

Bloody experts!

I was repeatedly asked by the experts: 'Does your speech gets worse when you're under stress?' My first thought was to understand what was meant by stress. Oh, no, something else to think about. I was told by the speech therapists: 'We're going to put you in these different situations and understand what gives you the most stress. Then we can make sure you have a coping mechanism.' I thought, *what's a coping mechanism?* I was now thinking about stress and coping mechanisms. I was often sent with other kids (or on my own) to a shop to buy sweets, or asked to role play to create a stressful situation. Sometimes I stuttered, sometimes I didn't. It wasn't helping. There was never a pattern.

I was now missing school for at least half a day to a day a week. I needed to travel on a bus to get to a hospital appointment. I would have the treatment and then travel back to school. Realistically, in a school day of 9:00 a.m. to 3:30 p.m., I could miss a whole day. Not only did I have a stutter, I was attending less and less school, causing me to fall behind with schoolwork. The voice in my head was starting to say, *you are now living proof that you're stupid.*

A glimmer of hope

I did meet some very perceptive people in the NHS. One speech therapist said, 'I don't think there is anything psychologically wrong with you. Your speech is not linked to any cause of anxiety that I can see.' But she did say: 'You are brave. You seem to hurtle to the edge of a cliff. But you have a habit of wanting to jump off. We call this self-sabotage.' Her view that I was not anxious gave some hope that I could be OK. Her insight on my self-sabotage was something that did live with me in a real way, well into my later life.

Nail varnish to make you sick

The increased self-awareness and growing self-doubt may have caused me to start biting my nails. I went through a period where my mum would paint this awful nail varnish stuff on to my nails. It tasted like crap and made me feel sick when I bit my nails. It also looked like I was wearing girls' nail varnish, which in 1974, unless you were a pop star like David Bowie, looked out of place. It didn't stop me biting my nails.

Stick this in your ears

The Edinburgh Masker was a new invention to help people who stuttered. You plugged a machine into your ears. When you spoke, it activated a very loud noise. The theory being, if you couldn't hear yourself speak, you would be able to talk without stuttering. I was on my way to the hospital with the contraption plugged in. A little old lady who was sitting next to me on the bus asked me if I knew when the stop for the hospital was. I didn't quite hear her question. So I asked her to repeat it. I couldn't hear myself or her speak as she spoke at the same time as me and the machine kicked in with a loud noise in my ears. I tried a couple of times to listen to what she was saying but it was hopeless. I still bloody stuttered. I looked and sounded like an utter freak. I was so frustrated! It didn't work for me! Maybe I didn't want it to either! I'm not a freak. I just can't speak.

All too much

All of the help, the advice from the experts, the pressure from my parents, life at school and the voices in my head were building. It was like a pressure cooker inside my head. At some point something had to give.

My mum and dad had a small touring caravan and would travel to different places around the UK, where we would stop for a few days or weeks during school holidays. My mum and dad would unhitch the caravan and manoeuvre it onto the pitch and set it up with gas and electricity. David (my younger brother) and I were shooed off, to go and explore the facilities and find other kids to play with. Caravanning was a very sociable activity. I quickly made short-term friends. I always found it liberating when we first arrived in a new place. We would explore the campsite, find the shop and go and play. All you needed was a football. However, the monkey on my back was never far away. The block in my throat. The thorn in my side. My stutter was always lurking below the surface. Waiting for an opportunity to make an unwanted appearance. But for a short time, I could just play football and hang out.

Life at school was difficult and at 14 years of age my anxiety levels were through the roof. I was getting stuck more often, unable to speak. Increasingly, I couldn't sleep. My mind was so active and the voices so loud – it could be unbearable. I would worry and focus on the smallest of things, like the origin of words. Why was the word red, red? Where did the word red come from? I became obsessed with what people thought of me and trying not to look stupid. I would try to insert words into a sentence that made me less likely to stutter. One voice would say, *should I speak or should I not speak?* on and on and on. It was relentless. It was like having a roundabout of thoughts racing round and round in your head. It would spin and spin and make me dizzy; it would spin faster and faster and was exhausting.

Parents have struggles too

My mum had so many issues with her own mum. She was one of five daughters and as a child was often ill. Her parents moved from Liverpool to London so she could be treated for respiratory problems and attend an open-air school. My mum never felt loved by her mum and believed she was the black sheep of the family. This was exacerbated when she and my dad moved from Liverpool to Billinge to set up their new home. The perceived lack of love caused my mum to get very upset. This became an issue for me when we were on holiday.

Nowhere to hide

My mum and dad would go out with friends to a local pub. Have a good time, and return for a late-night sandwich at one of the caravans. In a touring caravan all the beds are in the same small space. You can hear everything being said. My mum would get very upset and vocal. My dad was on holiday. He just wanted a few beers and a good time. They often ended up in huge rows about my mum's feelings about her mum. There was no hiding place, even when they tried to hide their fallout. The level of anger and upset really affected me. Were my parents going to get divorced? Why was my mum so unhappy? Was my nan so bad? The pressure cooker of being in the caravan intensified all these feelings and anxiety. The obsessive thinking, the overanalysis and the spinning in my head would get worse and worse. Of course, at 14 things can seem worse than they really are. And I was 14.

Medication, really?

I was on medication to reduce anxiety and help my stutter. One evening after a very bad argument between my mum and dad in the caravan I was at a real low. My life felt really crap. My stutter was causing me real issues with the kids we had met at the caravan park. I had been teased since the day we had arrived. I was being mocked and called all sorts of names. My mum and dad had been rowing for many nights. I was just sick of it all. I felt very unhappy and for some unknown reason I decided to take a row of eight tablets of my medication. I'm not sure why. I just did!

Saved by the boat

The next day at Aberystwyth Beach, I pushed our little boat into the water. A big wave caught the boat and the hull hit me on the back of the head and knocked me out. I was rushed to hospital in an ambulance. I woke up a few hours later to some very stern faces and had a massive plum-sized bruise on my head. My head was throbbing and I was still slightly dazed as I watched the nurse check the monitors I was attached to.

A few hours later one of the nurses asked me if I could speak. A doctor came to see me and said, 'Your mum and dad are very worried about you. Firstly because of the accident, and second, you seem to have taken a large number of your tablets at once. Can you explain if this is true and if so why?'

I was unable to give him an answer. I just stayed quiet. My mum and dad came in and asked me the same question. I still said nothing. It turned out that the tablets were placebos.

I would be left with a bruise on the head from the accident but there was no harm done. The whole incident was a shock to us all. Now I really didn't like myself. I couldn't even explain what I had done to myself. Why had I taken the tablets? No idea! I just knew I felt shit. The incident was not mentioned again while we were holiday. We carried on as normal. It must have been a huge worry for my parents. A stupid action on my part. A week after we arrived home, I'd forgotten the incident. My dad got me in a room. Looked me straight in the eye and just said, 'Never do that again.' I didn't. We all moved on.

Under the needle

My poor parents kept on searching for a fix. Sometimes the treatments appeared extreme. They were also expensive. But they were just doing the best they could. I'm so grateful my parents cared enough and sacrificed the things they did to help me. I remember one day going to Liverpool with my dad to a place called Rodney Street. My dad didn't give much away. I met a very smooth-looking and smartly dressed doctor who asked questions about my speech (the questions were always the same). I was told to come for my first appointment next week. Driving home, my dad still didn't explain the real purpose of the appointment and what would happen when I went back next week. I was confused.

Armed with a map, five pounds for the train fare and half a day off school, I set off for Lime Street railway station in Liverpool. This was a great adventure. I wasn't really sure where I was going or what for. Liverpool seemed so big and daunting. I arrived at Rodney Street after a taking a few wrong turns. The very nice nurse took me to the treatment room and told me to take my clothes off except for my underpants. The treatment room had a medical bed with a single white sheet on it. Next to the bed was an electronic contraption with dials, switches and leads coming out of the front. It looked like a sophisticated car battery charger! None the wiser, I was asked to lie on my front. The nurse explained that the doctor would start by sticking needles into my back. He's going to do what?! I was turned over and they stuck needles in my chest and all over. They stuck needles in my head, in and near my ears and worst of all in my feet. OMG, what had my dad agreed to do? The needles in my feet really hurt. It was like a scene from a scary movie. Everyone knew what was happening except for me.

I'm bleeding?

The nurse said she would be back later. I was left alone for about 40 minutes. I was feeling increasingly relaxed. It felt like I was floating above the bed. I fell asleep. The nurse came back and removed the needles. On the way out of the clinic, I read the sign: Acupuncture Clinic, Rodney Street. What the hell was acupuncture? I headed back to Lime Street railway station feeling like Mr Floppy. All relaxed and at one with the world. An old lady tapped me on the shoulder and in a brilliant thick Liverpool accent said, 'Eh love, do yer realize, you've got blood spurting out yer ear?' A very small stream of blood was spurting out, just below my ear. I just held my finger over the hole and ran for the train. Acupuncture made me feel relaxed, but it didn't cure my stutter. So what next?

Don't finish my sentence!

You get a lot of unwanted help when you have a stutter. People love to finish your sentence or even complete a word. They believe they're being helpful. Bless them. Do they get it right? Maybe. Should they try? No! When I was young this was hugely frustrating. I used to shut down and just let them think they were right, if they were or weren't. As I got into my early teens, I would let them say what they wanted to say and finish my own sentence. They could've been right. But I was going to have my goddam say. I would continue to push myself until I said the word or sentence. Sometimes they would be walking away before I finished. My response was to tell them to 'get lost!' (or maybe worse). I knew what I wanted to say. And I was going to say it. No matter how long it took me or who was listening!

'You know what you can do?'

Having a stutter is like having a baby, everyone has an opinion on how to help you. You may have heard:

Stop. Take deep breaths. Calm down. Slow down. Let me help you. Are you trying to say start, steal, steep, street? Can you draw the word? Go for a little walk and try again. It doesn't matter. Oh, oh,

… um… let me ask someone else. Have you had that seen to? Were you asked to change your writing hand when you were little? Am I making you anxious? Is it groups? Is it…? Don't worry, it doesn't matter.

Yes, it bloody well does.

Your story questions

- What treatments did you have?
- Did any work?
- Have you ever been pushed to your limit?
- What happened?

The ups and downs of senior school

On the evening of 6 March 1978, I went to Birchley St Mary's Catholic Club in Billinge to an under-18 disco. I went with a girlfriend and left with the girl who would become my wife, best friend and soulmate. St Mary's under-18 disco was a really cool place and the centre of the universe on a Monday night for all the kids in the area. I loved loud music, its vibrancy and the energy of people dancing and having fun. I had an eye for the girls and spent more time with girls than boys. I found them easier to talk to. They seemed to listen and were less likely to take the piss out of my speech. On this particular night, I was talking in the entrance of the club when Olivia Newton-John walked in. Oh my god, she was bouncy, vivacious and beautiful. This girl I had just seen took my breath away.

This unknown girl passed me by and went inside to dance. I immediately asked people, who is that? Christine Matthews, she goes to St Peter's High School, she's 16 years of age and has an older boyfriend. Damn. I was absolutely smitten. The next day I found where she lived and plucked up the courage to go and knock on her front door. Now you need to remember that I have a stutter. I'm going to a strange house, with people I don't know, to ask a girl if she will go out with me. Normally a massive no-no. I didn't care. I had to talk to her! Stuff the stutter. But this had all the ingredients of a huge fail. I wasn't expecting…

Her family don't like Scousers?

After pacing outside her house for over an hour, I plucked up the courage to go to the front door and ring the bell. My pulse was racing and my heart pounding furiously in my chest. My new denim jacket and jeans felt tight and I felt very awkward. A girl that wasn't Christine answered the door.

'Yes?'

I tried, 'Is Chri… Chris…. Chris… Christ… Christine in?'

Her sister, I later found out, said, 'No, sorry she's out. Who should I say called?'

A voice in my head said, *not a chance. I can't say my name, that will be the end of me!* I blurted out, 'I w-w-w-w will call back later.' There's no way I was going to say my bloody name. She would never go out with me. I found out later that her family didn't like Scousers (Wiganers just don't!). So I was right not to give them any more ammunition. But would that prevent her from seeing me? No, thank god!

But I was besotted

I called back at the house the night after and we started to see each other. I can't remember a time in my life when I had been so happy. She was the brightest, funniest, strongest person I had ever met. She was the yin to my yang. From the moment we met, it was unbearable to be apart. Saying goodbye was a tortuous process. 'I'm going now; OK, see you; one more kiss; one more hug, I'm definitely going now. It's late. Ok, just one more kiss; mmm. One more hug. One more joke. You go, no you go, no you go, no you go.' It was never dull, and from day one it felt that we were meant to be together. Some people talk about soulmates. I'm certain from my experience, it's true. It was a feeling of utter connectedness to another person. I had found mine and so much more. I didn't know what love was at 15. Who does? But I knew that I didn't want to spend a minute more than I had to away from my new BFF.

Caught skipping school

I was so desperate to spend time with Christine that I didn't go to school. Unfortunately, I was caught. My head of year, Des Seabrook (a great man), saw me getting on a bus going away from the direction of the school with Christine (to go to her sister's house), when he knew I should have been going to school. I knew I was in trouble. Des phoned my parents. Later that night my dad gave me a blast of the Alex Ferguson (Manchester United's famous and most successful football manager) hairdryer treatment. I didn't do it again.

Did Dracula have a stutter?

In the final year of high school, the English department held auditions for a musical production of *The Dracula Spectacular* musical. This caused me a lot of self-reflection and analysis. I really wanted to audition for the main role. I had a very strong feeling that I wanted perform in front of an audience. A part of me was becomingly increasingly confident and self-assured. Something to do with my new girlfriend. Who didn't seem to notice or maybe care that I stuttered. I loved to entertain people and I wanted to be part of something that seemed important to the school. But the internal doubt and the feelings that I would really screw up and let myself and the school down due to my stutter were very strong. I nearly didn't audition. The thought of humiliation was very powerful. The peer group pressure and the doubt that I would not be successful in the role didn't help.

However, a number of teachers said, 'It's a no-brainer. You should have a go and audition.' I got the main role of Dracula and will be forever grateful to the great teachers who took a risk on a kid with a stutter! Rehearsals started straight away. There were lots of lines to learn, songs to sing and dance moves to practise.

Did he lose his voice too?

I lost my voice a week before opening night. I don't know if it was the pressure I put myself under. Or was it the combination of the musical, impending exams, the fact my dad didn't want me to do the show, or was I just unlucky? The school had invested weeks in the production. Tickets had been sold. A large cast had rehearsed and here was the stuttering lead, with no voice. OMG. More doubt, more anxiety and it was building.

Five days to go. No voice. Four days to go. Still, I had no voice. Three days to go and Mr Hardman, my English teacher, turned up at my house and took me to the doctor. Bless him, he tried to persuade the doctor to give me some special medicine. 'Surely actors can get hold of stuff to help them?' he said. The doctor laughed and we left empty-handed. Two days to go. No voice. I went into school to find a workaround. It was decided I would mime. Someone else would read my lines. I didn't have an understudy.

Fangtastic

I didn't stutter once. The show was a brilliant success. I had got my voice back the day before opening night. I would later reflect that playing a character could be a way to hide my stutter. But that wouldn't be the real me. I would be someone else. That didn't feel right. And not a price I was prepared to pay. My dad came to see the show on the last night and was impressed. I spoke, sang and danced for two hours, for four nights, without a stutter in sight. For one night he was proud. Not that he told me. But he took me and Christine for a cheeky beer at a local pub! Miracles do happen!

A lot going on at school

My attitude to my O levels and CSE exams at high school was mixed. I was missing a lot of school due to my continued hospital treatments. I was involved in the rehearsals for *Dracula*. I had been appointed the school's first-ever head boy (someone else saw more in me than I could see in myself). I had a new girlfriend who I was besotted with. I had a part-time job drumming in a workingmen's club on Saturday and Sunday nights. I had a new drum teacher, Russell Cauldwell, who was a cool dude and reminded me of a '60s hippy. I was the captain of both the school's rugby and football teams. I also played for the Orrell rugby and Birchley football clubs at the weekend and trained during the week. I was in the cross-country team and ran the 400 metres and the relay for the school. I had lots of great stuff to keep me entertained. I didn't really understand the importance of exams. Unbeknown to me, my dad had applied for apprenticeship placements in a number of factories which would require more time off from school to take entry tests and attend interviews.

Second life fail

There is no doubt that having a stutter disrupted my life at high school. Not only was I absent from school due to hospital appointments, there was a whole lot more going on. I didn't realize, at the time, the detrimental impact all this time away from school would have on my education and that it would reinforce my dad's belief that I just wasn't clever enough! The treatments were not going well. I didn't feel particularly good about myself. I clearly remember seeing all our exam results, names and grades posted on the main school noticeboard. I got four O levels and six CSEs. However, the number of passes and the grades were a disaster compared to that of my friends. Many of whom were going on to do A levels at Winstanley College (the home of the grammar school). Not me. My dad had already predicted that I wasn't bright enough for A levels and I should get a job. My teachers thought I was mad. They said I would catch up with my peers if I did A levels. It was not to be. I had proved my dad right. Not bright enough! Not good enough! Time to start work!

An end and a beginning

So that was my life till I left school at 17 years of age to start work as an apprentice. I don't want you to think that I was just an anxious wreck or completely negative about life because of my stutter. It was more complicated than that. I don't know how you feel about your stutter and how it affected you and your life at that age. At 17, I had many opposing and contrary feelings and voices in my head.

On the one hand, I was hugely optimistic about life. Even though I was going to do a job that I didn't understand or want to do. I felt smart in so many ways, even though the resounding voice in my head was saying I wasn't bright enough. On the one hand, I felt apprehensive about new situations, but at the same time I was hungry for adventure and excited to learn new things. I wanted to hide away, but at the same time I wanted to take on the world. I wanted to stay in my head and not speak, yet I had lots to say. I didn't know where I was going, but I knew I was going somewhere. I was going to have fun and I knew my life was going to be better than it was today. I always felt that I had something big to offer the world, without a clue what that meant. It was just a feeling. I still have those same feelings today. I can be more! Life is never black and white. It's shades of grey. But I knew I needed to follow my feelings of wanting to be more.

Your story questions

- How did you do at school?
- Was your education impacted by your stutter?
- Did you know what you wanted to do after school?
- What happened?

Starting work

I was employed as an electrical and electronics apprentice at BAE Systems, missile division, Lostock, just outside of Bolton in the north-west of England. The apprenticeship would last four years. The first year was an introduction to a wide range of technical skills, including electronic wiring and soldering, electronic testing and repair, milling, turning, toolmaking, CNC machining and a wide range of other skills to prepare us for the world of work. It sounds stupid, but I didn't have a clue what I was about to do and where it would lead. Other than the words of my dad ringing in my ears, 'You'll always have something to fall back on', whatever that meant! What on earth was I going to do with skills to fix missiles?

I would leave home at 5:30 a.m. to catch the bus outside Billinge Hospital to Wigan town centre. I would then walk across Wigan to catch the bus to the factory at Lostock to start work at 7:42 a.m. I was still undergoing a number of treatments for my stutter. But I could feel something changing in my head.

A life decision

At 17, I made a major life decision. Early on in my apprenticeship, my dad had arranged for me to see a hypnotherapist, another attempt to fix my stutter. I left work. Got a bus and went to the private wing of Wigan hospital. I had a consultation and I began my first hypnotherapy session. I was asked to relax and the process of hypnotherapy began.

I remember it was a beautiful sunny day when I left the clinic. I was happy. I had a job, I was earning money. I was playing drums at the weekend to earn extra money. I was fit and felt strong and learning a whole bunch of new stuff. I wasn't overly interested in work but it was something different. More importantly, I had a girlfriend that I was head over heels in love with. I decided on that day that I didn't need or want any more speech treatments. I decided I didn't want anyone else trying to find out what was wrong with me. And fix me. I didn't feel broken. I felt hugely optimistic about me. I wanted to get on with my life. I didn't want this constant, reinforced external doubt from others plaguing my life. I had enough doubt and anxiety in my own head without adding to the noise from other sources.

Stop the medical treatments!

I decided this was it. No more treatment. After making that decision, I remember feeling such a sense of relief. A letting go. A moving on. I just needed to tell my dad. It's difficult to remember his reaction all these years later, but I wasn't bothered at the time. It just felt like the right thing to do. Ultimately, my dad was only trying to help his son. I now had to help myself. There is only so much parents can do for you. At some point you have to make up your own mind up and forge your own way in the world. My mind was set. My stutter would not hold me back. It would not define who I was. I felt more than my stutter. I now had to push on and push through the stutter.

Gareth Gates, English pop singer and actor, said, 'Young adults living with a stutter is [sic] hard work. How do they handle job interviews? What do they do when the phone rings? How do they "chat someone up"? All these things the average person takes for granted prove to be a stammerer's biggest challenge.'[7]

Spin 'em and prove 'em

My apprentice training school had many quirks. The training rooms had old cast iron radiators that couldn't be turned off. In the middle of summer, the training rooms were stifling hot and the windows could only be opened slightly. Consequently, many of us were caught

---

[7] Gates, 'Gareth Gates – stop my stutter', n.d.

nodding off at some point during a training session. The penalty for sleeping could result in a loss of wages or suspension. The instructors knew it was hard to stay awake and revelled in catching us sleeping.

One day I was caught having a nice little nap while learning about Whitworth screw threads (I know, how could I? Ha!). Whitworth threads were enough to put anyone to sleep. After being woken up, I was escorted out of the classroom and told to report to the instructors' office in the morning. How was I going to get out of this? I came up with a story and went to see the head instructor and the instructor who had caught me asleep.

'Now, son, what happened yesterday?'

'Well,' I said, 'I have insomnia and I take tablets every day to keep me awake.' I showed them the bottle of tablets I had brought from home, without a label of course. I continued, 'I had run out of tablets that day. See the bottle? Hence, I fell asleep. It won't happen again.' This was a big deal for me. I didn't want a note on my record or, worse, a suspension. They both looked at each other and told me to get out and not fall asleep again. Phew!

You lucky git!

I went back to the electronics training room.

My mates were buzzing. 'What happened? Have you been suspended?'

'No, they let me off.' I told them the insomnia story which the instructors had believed. We all laughed and enjoyed the moment.

The electronics instructor came back into the room just as I was finishing the story. He said, 'I would like a word in your shell-like, Mr Gaskin!'

David Tongue, like many of the instructors, had his own little phrases. He told me that the instructors hadn't believed a word of the insomnia story. He went on to say that they had heard many a cock and bull story in their lives. But it was the first time they had ever heard *that* cock and bull story. As a result, they let me off.

Electrified electronics instructor!

Getting into trouble was becoming an unwanted but regular event. This was not helping the voices in my head or my stutter. On another occasion, the electronics instructor got a severe electric shock while wiring up a circuit board, much to the amusement of the class of apprentices. I thought I would write up the incident in my weekly logbook. I drew a picture of the instructor with an electric shock going through his body, as a reminder of how dangerous electricity could be. He did not find my picture of him being electrocuted amusing at all. He thought I had showed a complete lack of respect. I was sent to the head instructor to explain my actions. He made me sweat for a whole week before letting me know whether I would lose my job. Shit, shit, what would my dad say to me? I really didn't like what I was doing. But I didn't want the embarrassment of being kicked out of the apprenticeship programme. Friday arrived. I was wheeled in to what felt like a court martial.

The head instructor looked again at the picture, smiled, and said, 'Fancy yer self as a bit of a Van Gogh, do yer?'

'N-n-n-n-n-n-no,' I stuttered. That's when the tightening of the throat happens, the clicking of the tongue, the sweaty palms and the lack of oxygen to the brain. I literally felt like I was going to pass out. 'It was not meant to be f-f-f-f-f-f-f-funny,' I said, 'it was just a picture of w-w-w-w-w-w-what, happened.'

He closed the book, smiled, and said, 'He can be a bit sensitive, can David [the instructor]. Mind how you go, lad, you've had too many warnings from me. This will be your last.'

Thank god for that! I left, telling myself to keep my nose clean and focus on what I was doing.

Off the bus on to two wheels

In hindsight, my dad was making me do the basics to prepare for life. He forced me to get a job, to learn skills and earn money. So no matter what happened later in life, as he said, I would have something to fall back on. He also taught me how to get and pay back loans from the bank. After going to work on the bus, he decided that I needed to take my motorbike test. But first I needed a motorbike. We went to Rogersons, the local motorbike shop, where I bought a Honda 100 (a 100-cc motorbike). I got a loan which I would pay back over a three-year period. I enrolled in a motorbike school at weekends, where I had to pass their test before I could take the real Department of Transport test. It worked. On a snowy day in January 1980, when I was 18, I passed my motorbike test. First time.

A mini adventure

After passing my motorbike test I wanted to buy a more powerful motorbike, a Honda Dream (a 250-cc motorbike), but the insurance was scandalous for an 18-year-old. I bought a car; it was much cheaper and kept me dry. I bought a Mini® Traveller, 1968. It cost me GBP 300. I sold the motorbike and paid off my loan. Christine called the car Betsy. We rubbed down the wood on the back of the car, varnished it and bought new blue carpet from a shop in Billinge. Betsy was my pride and joy. We bought a plastic cover to put over the distributor cap and spark plugs. This would keep them dry, so the car wouldn't stop when it rained. The quirky car also needed you to turn the heater on full blast on a long journey or the engine would overheat. The heaters would fry your feet. But we loved it! I now just had to pass my driving test.

I can't tell my left from my right

I passed my driving test on 23 June 1980 in Wigan. I had learned to drive in my uncle's Vauxhall® Victor, a big green car. My dad and I had fallen out big time while he was teaching me. You didn't pay for lessons back then. They were too expensive. He would shout and chastise me for getting things wrong, which, to be fair, was often. There was no dual control in the Vauxhall® Victor. On a number of occasions, I nearly crashed the car, or at least it felt like that. Hey ho. Who said life was easy?

Finally, the day of the driving test arrived. Unfortunately, the car I was taught in was not available. I had to take the Mini® I had recently bought, which I was pretty unfamiliar with and had only driven a couple of times. At the test centre, the biggest driving examiner you could ever imagine got into my little Mini®. He was so big that I couldn't easily put the car into gear due to his big legs encroaching on my side of the car and blocking the gear stick. I checked my mirror and pulled out of the test centre. Easy does it, I thought. I was very aware of this huge presence next to me with his big beard and a stern look on his face. At the end the road was a one-way system. I made the left turn. The test had begun.

Third life fail averted!

The most difficult part of the test, other than parallel parking, was the navigation of the Beech Hill housing estate – a warren of roads that were not clearly marked. I also had another affliction, other than my stutter. I can't tell my left from my right (I haven't mentioned my partial dyslexia yet). Twice, I was heading off the Beech Hill estate, and twice, the examiner said take the next left. Twice, I turned right and took the wrong turn. Bummer, I thought that's it, I'll not pass now. On the way back to the test centre, another learner driver was in trouble, as she was failing to complete her three-point turn. I stopped the car and waited patiently for her to complete her manoeuvre. I thought I had already failed my test. So I thought best I wait and give her a fighting chance. Later I found out that this had been the correct decision.

Sharp those brakes

The final part of the driving test was the emergency stop. The driving examiner said, 'When I bring my clipboard down on the dashboard, stop the car.' A few minutes later, I noticed, out the corner of my eye, that he had started to move his clipboard down. I anticipated the instruction and slammed on the brakes. The car shuddered to a stop. The poor examiner hurtled towards the windscreen. There were no self-adjusting seatbelts in an old Mini®. He got a real jarring in his seat. And his head just hit the windscreen.

A little winded, he said, 'Sharp those brakes, lad!'

I nodded and carried on back to the test centre. I was convinced I had failed. But to my surprise, I only had one minor observation and I had passed. First time. I could now use my car to drive to work and college.

Your story questions

- How did your stutter impact getting and doing your first job?
- What was your first experience of work like?
- Have you ever made any big decisions about your stutter?

College catastrophes

In the first year of my apprenticeship I was enrolled on a Business, Technology, Education Course (BTEC), Ordinary National Certificate (ONC). My first lecture was maths. The lecturer, Mr Nutall, walked in and shouted gruffly, 'I always get the "thickies" from BAE.'

I don't know why. I saw the red mist. I was on my feet, infuriated. 'Who are you calling a thickie?' I had a temper back then. The rest of the class just laughed at me. The next hour was painful. It was so low level.

To be fair, Mr Nutall came up to me at the end of the lesson. He apologized and said, 'I can see you're smarter than this programme son. You need to go and see Rob Brewer, head of the Higher National Certificate and Diploma programmes.'

Rob to the rescue

When I met Rob, I was still quite angry. I was on an apprenticeship programme I didn't want to do. In a class with people I didn't want to be with. I was bored and I felt humiliated at the level of the course I was on. Another year of this? I don't think so! Rob was a super guy. We chatted. He listened and asked me about my O Level and CSE grades. After a discussion he said, 'Lad, you're too bright for this programme. I will ring the BAE Training School and get you on the Higher National Certificate (HNC) programme.' He did. The next week I was transferred and started a programme that at least got my brain going. I passed the HNC with flying colours. The result persuaded the training school to put me on the Higher National Diploma Programme (HND) in Microelectronics and Communications. Thank you, Rob. Like many others in my career, you spotted something in me that was worth a punt. Most importantly, you did something practical to help!

I hated the first day of anything

It was the first day of the two-year Higher National Development (HND) course. I was in a class of 20 students from different companies. As with every other lesson in every other school, college or university around the world, they would start with the registration. In this case, Dr Kitt Latham said, 'OK, around the room, give me your name and the company you work for.' I know what you're thinking. How hard can that be? Unless you, the reader, has a stutter. Right?

The night before my new HND course would start, I knew that the first day would be a nightmare. A day of saying, or in my case, not saying, my name. That sinking feeling in my stomach was horrible. Trying to relax, trying to stay positive, trying not to care, trying to put it to the back of my mind, thinking of strategies to get me to say Paul Gaskin. How hard could that be? The voices in my head were at work and ready to get turbocharged. Roll the dice.

Could it be easier this year?

Driving to college with my radio on. The voices in my head had started. *Maybe I would make a joke before trying to say my name. That had worked before. Maybe I would use some of my old techniques. I could say when asked, say, Aul Gasin and miss out the P and the K. That's always a bit easier. Maybe I could get someone else to say my name. How embarrassing would that be? I could have a quiet word with the lecturer?* I arrived at college and parked my car and went to the canteen. I was the joker. I liked to talk. I liked the banter. I didn't like to say my name. I had learned to say what I wanted to say by being funny. I also used humour to remove, as best I could, the embarrassment other people would feel when I started to stutter. I had used many techniques in prior years in college, but it was not getting any easier, in some ways. Because I now felt I had to prove myself in a higher quality class of student, the potential embarrassment felt greater.

Count down to the dreaded question

The college day began. We strolled into the classroom and found our seats. I would always sit at the back. This would give me the maximum time to prepare, to breathe slowly, think of funny things to distract the class. I could have some banter with the guy next to me and relax myself. I looked around the room and noticed what was going on. The lecturer had started. Eight people to go before I have to say my name. The voice in my head starts: *Just say your name under your breath. Paul Gaskin. My name is Paul Gaskin.* Seven people to go. The voice: *Sit up straight, breathe.* My throat is feeling tight. Can I get some water? Six people to go. I whisper to Steve, the guy next to me, 'Can you say my name for me?'

'No,' he says.

They're moving more quickly through the names now. They are so nonchalant. The voice in my head: *Listen to him,* 'My name is Mark and I am from blah blah', *so easy for him to say, piss off!* Five more to go. The voice in my head: *This is going to be shit, stand up it's easier to breathe. No, sit down you will look a prat.* Four more to go. My mind is racing. *Should I insert a word? Should I say my name is Alan? No, no you can't do that when they find out they will think you're an arse. I hate this, how many years have I been doing this?* My mind goes into a tailspin. *How hard can it be?* My throat is tighter. Three more to go. It's the guy on the next table. Other people in the class are turning around to see who is speaking. The voice in my head is saying, *please don't turn around. This will be a car crash. I'm tired and that will make it worse. I should have gone to bed earlier. I should have got up and gone for a run early this morning; that normally helps.* Two people to go. I can hear my heart pounding in my chest. *Insert a word. Say a joke. Call out something. OMG, why is this so difficult. Do I really need to be here?*

Have you not said your name yet?

Why am I putting myself through this bloody pain? I need to find a different approach. One more to go before me. My throat is now tight as hell. I'm trying to breathe. *Stand up. It's easier when you stand up. Oh no, it's me.* Dr Kitt Latham looks at me expectantly, pen poised over the register. 'P-P-P-P-P-P-P, my name is P-P-P-P-P... P-P-P-P-P-P-P-P-P.' My neck is so tight. I'm biting my tongue and pushing it against my teeth. I'm making a clicking noise in my throat. The voice in my head is saying, *can other people hear that clicking?* The lecturer now looks embarrassed and wants to help. Someone says something. *Was it aimed at me? I will kick their head in, if they're taking the piss?* I feel sorry for the lecturer. He only wants my name. 'P-P-P-P-P-P... P-P-P-P-P-P-P-P-P-P-P'. I'm not going to stop. My head feels lighter and I'm getting really frustrated. 'Oh bollocks!' I say out loud. 'Sorry, I can never say my bloody name. It's P-P-P-P-P... P-P-P-P-P-P-P-P-P.' I then say out loud, 'Wait, it's coming.' And the lecturer looks even more confused. The voice in my head says, *Dr Kitt Latham thinks I'm winding him up.* Deep breath. 'My name is P-P-P-P-P-P-Paul Gaskin, my name is P-P-P-P-Paul Gaskin,' I blurt. 'Shit, I'm so sorry that it is just so hard.' I had noticed that everyone in the room had looked so tense. The class relaxes. Everyone is relieved; my name is out of the way! Until the next class!

It's so exhausting

It's so hard to explain how loud and fast the voices in my head are travelling when all this is going on. It's like an express train screaming down a track. At the end of saying my name, I'm absolutely exhausted. And this is the first class of a day that starts at 9:00 a.m. and ends at 8: 30 p.m. Of course, the same thing happened every year and on every course I ever went on throughout my 40-year career.

'People only stutter at the beginning of the word. They're not afraid when they get to the end of the word. There's just regret.'[8] This quote from Laurie Anderson, American avant-garde composer, musician and film director, represents something that is hard to explain to a non-stutterer. The self-reflection and mental trauma (I don't use this word lightly) and anguish caused can be unbearable. You can go over and over what you've just said. The horrible feelings you felt and feel. And how you think you made others feel. It can take days to get over a bad episode.

As Joseph G. Sheehan said, 'Stuttering is like an iceberg, with only a small part above the waterline and a much bigger part below.'[9] It's so bloody true!

Your story questions

- Do you have problems saying your name?
- How do you get through those situations?
- How does it make you feel?

---

8 Krasuski, 'Regret avoidance', 2019.
9 Sheehan, *Stuttering: Research and Therapy*, 1970.

Do you care about what others think?

Working in a factory was tough

Life at college compared to working on the shop floor was a breeze!

After the first year of my apprenticeship in the underground training school, I was moved to West Block (part of the main factory complex), where missiles of all types and sizes were manufactured, assembled and tested. I was to be taught how to wire and test missiles. The factory was located in Lostock in Bolton, which is nearer to Manchester than to Liverpool. Unbeknown to me at that time, there is a built-in dislike of Scousers if you are from Bolton (as in Wigan). So I was caught completely off guard, when after a couple of days working on the Skyflash missile assembly line, I heard there was a Scouser in West Block. Who might that be, I thought? I never thought it was me! Although I'm very proud to have been born in Liverpool, it never occurred to me that other people would see me as a Scouser. I didn't have a strong accent. I hadn't lived in Liverpool since I was three years of age. No matter, to other people I still wore the badge.

They really don't like Scousers?

To my utter amazement, people would come from all over West Block and other parts of the factory to take the piss out of the Scouser. And to be honest, it could be surprisingly aggressive. I would be ridiculed for the performance of the Liverpool football team and subjected to a whole range of jokes. Too many to mention, but typically they would start with, 'What do you call a Scouser in a suit? The accused, ha.' Followed by, 'Piss off, you Scouse git,' (I've toned down the language used in a factory to spare both our blushes) for absolutely no rhyme or reason that I could fathom. 'What do you call a Scouser in a house? A burglar.' The jokes were a lot worse than these tame examples. It could be intense. At times, the verbal abuse would escalate, and at times, it would get physical. There was a stream of men in my face, fuelled with anger and resentment that I didn't understand. I was genuinely shocked. I would respond to their tirades, and OMG, it would appear. My mate. My stutter. There for the attackers to ridicule. My stutter caused derision and utter contempt. A flaw. A fault. Another reason for a personal attack had surfaced. 'Ha ha, you freak, a s-s-s-s-s-s-stuttering S-S-S-S-S-S-Scouser. You are a useless stupid, stuttering Scouse git. Aren't you?' My stutter was ammunition for their AK-47s.

What the hell do I do now?

For a few weeks I really was taken aback and went into a spiral of self-reflection and hurt. While outwardly not giving an inch. I didn't want to go to work. I didn't want to tell my dad. I could hear his answer, 'Son, stand up and be counted. No excuses, you don't back down!' So I didn't. I made a decision. Stuff them all. They would get abuse back and more than they could handle. They wanted a fight? They were going to get one. Prepare the missiles!

Step up born-again Scouser

I started to learn a lot more about the Liverpool Football Club. Players, history, trophies and getting as many facts as I could. Part of my ammunition to fight back. I also learned about their teams. Manchester United and the local team Bolton Wanderers. More than that. I had decided that I was going to make a stand. I decided that if anyone had a go at me, no matter who it was, or at whatever level in the organization, I was going to have a right old go back. I had a phrase that I would use when people started attacking me, which served me well. My mantra for many years was like a speech before a fight. 'You can start if you want? But I will finish it. Do you want to start?' Unfortunately, for most people, I was quicker, more sarcastic, more cutting and prepared to push the boundaries of what most people wanted to say. I had created a no holds barred monster to defend myself. I had a fire in my belly. But this fire and desire to stand up for myself felt different. It was personal. I became a lot more aggressive and mentally tough in a surprisingly short amount of time.

Where is this all going?

I have to say that most of the people on the shop floor were brilliant. We had good banter most of the day, but some of the attacks were not friendly banter. Today it would be called bullying or harassment. But for me it became character defining. Sink or swim? Bring it on!

During the next few weeks things turned bitter as I pushed back. Some people walked away. Others wanted to fight. Swearing. Finger pointing, raised voices and pushing became more the norm. The downside of me pushing back was all the unwanted attention. This wasn't appreciated by the chargehand and the foreman (the supervisors), who now had a nuclear weapon on their assembly line. I was just a nuisance disrupting their equilibrium.

Now what? You want a fight?

One apprentice came down for some banter that went too far. He just couldn't take or respond to my very hurtful comments about him. He lost his temper and said, 'I'll get you tomorrow at college. Me and my mates are going to kick the hell out of you. You stuttering Scouse git.' *Yikes*, I thought to myself, *now what do I do*?

The next morning, I arrived at college at 8:45 a.m. On time for my 9:00 a.m. lesson. The abusive apprentice was at the gate with four of his mates. They blocked my path and jostled me as I pushed through.

'You're going to be a dead Scouser,' his mates said. 'At break we will take you to the post office and kick the shit out of you.'

In my head I thought, *why the post office*? I was worried. Five of them? I'll take them all on. But they're not great odds. I could get my head kicked in here. What the hell do I do now?

Decision time – he's in the canteen on his own

Part way through the first lesson. Unusually, I went to the canteen to buy a cup of tea and a Mars® bar. The abusive apprentice stood in front of me and was without his mates. I said, 'Let's do this now!'

He said, 'Fine, let's go to the post office.' I was still clueless as to why we were going to the post office. As we walked out of college, I was thinking *shit, this could end really badly. I could get thrown off the HND course for fighting.* The voices in my head were starting. *Did he have a knife? How do you start a fight?* My previous fights had only ever been playing sport.

After 10 minutes we arrived at the post office in Wigan Town Centre. (I was still none the wiser.) I said to him, 'How do you start the fight?' He said he would say 'right' and we would start. But before he got to the 't', I just punched him a number of times in the face. I think it was just the adrenaline. I didn't really want to fight. I wanted to get back to college. I was so worried about the consequences of what we were doing. Playing hard at rugby and tackling is not the same as a street fight.

Are they dimples on your face?

I'd thrown a few very quick, powerful and accurate punches and caught him completely by surprise. Stunned, he wrestled me to the floor. Now I really didn't know what to do. He was just clinging on and not really doing anything. An old grizzly Wiganer poked me with his walking stick and said, 'Get on you boys, or I will call the police.'

Yikes, I thought. I said to the abusive apprentice who was still clinging on for dear life. 'This is stupid, let's go.' We got up and as I looked at him, I noticed square marks on his face where my ring had caught him. Christine, my beautiful girlfriend, had bought me a square-shaped gold ring set with a green onyx head for my birthday. The Elizabeth Arden range (Argos, they were the rage at the time). I was so in love with Christine that I always wore it on my wedding finger. I liked to flick the onyx head with my finger. So much so, that one day the green onyx popped out and I lost it. Such was my embarrassment that I kept wearing the ring. It was now a gold ring with a square empty space, where the green onyx head had once been. The empty space left by the lost onyx had created square-shaped dimples on his face. Doh!

I didn't feel great at all. This was bloody stupid! I said, 'That's it, I'm going back to college.' I spent a whole day agonizing about the potential repercussions. If he reported me to the training school, or worse, to the police, I would lose my job!

Shake hands and move on

The next day in work, I went and found the guy to make sure he was all right. I apologized, and said, 'Let's shake hands and crack on'. He agreed and no more was said. That's what I liked about blokes, well, in years gone by. Have a bust-up. Even a fight. Next day, it's all forgotten. His face still looked like he had been hit with a little hammer.

Unpacking complex feelings

I didn't really want to fight anyone. But I wanted to fight everyone! I didn't want to be pushed around or threatened. Was that my dad's voice or was it mine? I felt strong and brave. But I also felt frightened. One voice was saying, *it's time to make a stand*. Another said, *let it go*. Runaway! I took charge of the situation to make sure I had a chance in the fight. In my head I won. But why did I feel like I'd lost? I felt shame, not glory. I wanted peace. Not further conflict. So I made amends.

Making a stand for me!

To fight was a tough decision. On reflection and hypothetically, I had a choice to fight or not to fight, but in my mind, it wasn't really a choice. He and his mates wanted blood and they had the better odds. The decision to take on one was better odds than taking on five. That was my rationale. Fighting is never the right answer. But sometimes it's a necessary answer. Word got around the factory. You can take on the Scouser, but he's not scared to fight you! This felt like my voice! I was making a stand for me. The constant abuse stopped overnight. Equilibrium on the assembly line was restored. This felt like another turning point in my life. And it was.

Your story questions

- Has your stutter ever got you into trouble?
- What was the situation and what happened?
- Have you ever decided to stand up for yourself?
- What other experiences have shaped your character?

Singing on the shop floor: what could possibly go wrong?

Life on the shop floor was always full of unexpected and unpredictable events.

West Block became a place where I was learning new skills and having my eyes opened about life. The first floor of West Block employed a few hundred women and some men in wiring, assembling and testing missiles. Women were employed as semi-skilled labour primarily to wire the missiles, as they were typically more dexterous and quicker than men. As I learned, women could wire the missiles, talk and take the piss all day. The few men who worked on the assembly line knew in no uncertain terms who was in charge.

The women sat on long work benches arranged in rows. Each part of the missile assembly process was laid out from the front to the back of the factory floor. The floor had a chargehand and a foreman who made sure that work was delivered on time. Apprentices were fair game for the women and part of their daily sport. It was largely good banter full of innuendo which they used to pass the time.

Who's up for a Christmas carol?

I was told that apprentices could make a lot of money from carol singing. I was in my second year and earned GBP 45 per week. The older apprentices said you could earn up to GBP 20 for a couple of songs. Very handy at Christmas.

There were about 15 apprentices working on the assembly line. We were given song sheets and told to stand in the middle of the shop floor away from the benches. Most of the lads were pretty fit. We played rugby, football or, like myself, did martial arts or some other form of physical activity like weight training. We were between the ages of 19 and 21. We all thought we were pretty handy and would fight anyone. How the mighty fall!

Anyone who has a stutter will tell you they can sing without stuttering. It's brilliant and liberating. We started to sing our first song: 'Oh Come, All Ye Faithful'. The women had downed their tools and seemed to be listening. At the start of the second song, as I looked around the audience, I could see cans of lager being distributed. Now this was a clean area. You couldn't have any food or drink as it would contaminate the assembly process. I also noticed a group of women moving from their benches towards us. As we started 'Good King Wenceslas', the women were saying to each other 'rip their clothes off' (I noticed everything that went on around me. One benefit of having a stutter, you play close attention to others, when they speak). *Do what?* I thought. Rip their clothes off! I could see them mouthing that to each other. This must be a joke. Banter? Even if they did try, they couldn't. There are 15 of us. How wrong can one young man be?

Good king HelpLESSness!

A sudden flash and flurry. The women, who knows how many, pounced from the front and the back and started to rip our clothes off in a very rough, no-nonsense way. The 1980s were obviously different times. It wasn't a great experience. Not for us! It was very physical with hands and fingers everywhere they shouldn't have been. I was scratched, bitten and pinched, and we ended in less clothes than we had come to work in, and having our backsides slapped down the shop floor. The place had gone mad. I could hear shouts, screams and banshee-type noises. Lots of women shouting at us, describing our bodies and what they would do to us. Lots of laughing and singing. Suck it up. All banter and part of the fun. Their fun! The Christmas festivities had begun.

We were black and blue

I got home that evening. I was very bruised, not only from the slapping and pinching, but also my ego had taken a bit of a hiding as well. I was black, blue, purple and a whole range of other none-normal skin colours. On the one hand, it was part of the apprentice induction and an interesting insight into the power of the fairer sex. They were very generous for their entertainment and we made GBP 25 each. I was a little humbler walking back on the shop floor after Christmas. A little more respectful of the women I worked with. It was all part of the banter of working on the shop floor. Behind the perfume, the lipstick and the hairspray lay a toughness and a no-nonsense steel. Many of the women were working to bring up families. Some were single parents. Most were just trying to better themselves and their families. I saw many men underestimate them during my years on the shop floor. There was only ever one winner.

Who is making that sucking noise?

In the last year of my year apprenticeship, I was awarded Apprentice of the Year and attended a big event to receive my award from the company CEO. I had completed a four-year apprenticeship in two years. To keep me stimulated and, I'm sure, out of trouble, I was moved to other parts of the factory, where the engineering apprentices were trained on their rotations. I'd successfully transferred to the technical apprentice course and successfully passed my Higher National Diploma in Microelectronics and Communications with distinction. I would take on any task or project, and had a reputation for getting things done.

My dad and Christine attended the awards event. My dad was being his normal irreverent self. Every time he saw me talking to someone in a suit (a boss in his words), he would make a sucking noise and say, 'You little suck-up, who's a suck-up.' He really didn't care. I just ignored him and got on with it. I knew by then that this was just my dad taking the mickey out of me. He was telling me, in his own way, 'don't get too big for your boots.' No matter what I did. Parental banter with edge. I remember that in my 18th birthday card he had written in brackets after 'Happy Birthday' – 'don't get too big for your boots!' It was my dad's way of trying to keep me grounded. He didn't realize that I was doing a pretty good job of that all by myself.

Your story questions

- What has work been like for you?
- Have you encountered any bullying?
- What did you learn about yourself?
- What did you do?

Part 2

Your life, using the lessons learned

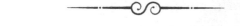

Get ready to change your life

The next part of the book is all about you. Your life story and using the lessons learned from my life to become so much more than your stutter. It will be helpful to have your Success Workbook (journal) ready to record your responses to the exercises, questions and your learning. I want to share with you the book that changed my life, how to manage the voices in your head and an overview of the five-step process you will use to change your life.

The book that changed my life

In my early 20s I read a book called *The 4%* by Dr Kushel, an American educator and author. Dr Kushel interviewed 500 senior leaders from the top Fortune 500 companies in the USA to find out if they were happy with their work, with their family life and with themselves. He found that only 4% of the people he interviewed were happy in all three areas. Most were only happy in one area, sacrificing at least one or maybe both the other areas, which was normally their family and themselves. I wanted to be happy in all three. I found the book a call to action for what I wanted my life to be.

What did the 4% know?

Dr Kushel's research showed that people in the 4% had some common characteristics. They knew life was unfair, they knew it was finite and that they alone were responsible for how they felt. The 4% knew it was down to them to design and live their lives, and to decide how they would respond to whatever happened to them. He said they all had a mental image of themselves that was bigger than themselves and linked to nature. Dr Kushel went on to describe a simple process of planning and designing a life that changed my life.

The reading of *The 4%* started me on a track of reading self-help books and seeking out ways to become a better version of me. It surfaced strong feelings and a real desire to live a balanced life. To be comfortable in my own skin, have a happy and loving family life, great friends, to find work that I truly believed had purpose, to be excited and enjoy life. Ultimately, I wanted to be happy and contented with myself. But happy and contented meant I needed to push myself to be so much more than I was at that point in my life.

Your version of the 4%

I'm hoping that the next part of the book becomes a catalyst for you and your life, as *The 4%* was for me. You've already got a lot of life experiences. You know about you. You know some of the things you want from your life. You will know some of the things you're good at and want to do more of. You will also know how you like to learn. And what works and doesn't work for you. I want you to read the next part of the book applying your experiences and your ambitions to the exercises we're about to do. Keep asking yourself, how will this work for me?

Your thoughts determine your life

In the first part of the book, I spoke a lot about the voices in my head. I don't know if you've had a similar experience. To be honest, until I was given a book in my late 20s, titled *What to Say When You Talk to Yourself* by Shad Helmstetter, I thought I was odd. Then I understood. Everyone has a voice or voices in their head. The voices are your thoughts. Your thoughts determine how you feel. How you feel determines what you do. Ultimately, what you do determines the life you have.

As far back as 1637, Descartes wrote, 'I think, therefore I am'.[10] Since then, the five reputed fathers of psychology, Sigmund Freud, Carl Jung, William James, Ivan Pavlov and Alfred Alder, and in the present day, John R. Anderson, Dan Ariely and Elliot Aronson, have all researched and commented on the link between thinking and doing (behaviour). I have personally learned a lot from modern psychology, neuroscience and self-help authors including Joe Dispenza, Tony Robbins and many others who are focused on making psychological concepts accessible and practical.

How do they do that?

Your thoughts are the result of your experiences and how you make sense of them. These experiences start from when you are born. Therefore, your parents have a huge impact on what you think and what you now do, as do your friends, teachers, the media and the world around you. You take in information, then you interpret what it means for you. That determines how you feel and that in turn determines what you do. For example, my parents tell me stealing is bad. I think their thought, stealing is bad. I want to feel good by pleasing my parents. I don't steal. Not only do I not steal in that moment, but that thought and feeling is now programmed into me and becomes just what I do. I don't steal. I'm simplifying a complex interaction of what goes on in your head, your processing and therefore what you do. But you get the idea, right? Think, feel, do, repeat.

By the time you become a young adult, much of what you think, feel and do is automatic. You see or hear something, you get an automatic

---

[10] Descartes and Cress, *Discourse on Method (Third Edition)*, 1998.

feeling and you take action. It's like breathing. You don't think about it. Have you ever heard someone say, 'I always do that'? Or they may say, 'I don't know why I do that'? Or they have a belief about something, but they don't know why?

You'll have thoughts and feelings about your stutter. What you can and can't do and how you feel about yourself (largely from what others have told you, especially if they were negative). You'll also have voices in your head about a whole range of other things, again, mainly from parents. Mine would say things like 'nothing is worth having unless it's hard to do; don't look down on people; you need to get a job, not A levels'. But they would also say positive things. Unfortunately, the positives can get lost in the noise. Even simple things like saying to you, 'be careful'; as a child, you can interpret this as 'avoid taking a chance'. So when you become a young adult, you may not want to take many chances that may feel like a risk.

So what?

The voices of others, and the experiences of your life so far, have likely caused you to think the way you do today. The thoughts you have today will determine what you do and don't do today. I know from my own experiences, I wouldn't have had the life I have lived, if I had only listened to the voices my parents put in my head. My dad wouldn't speak to me for two weeks when I left BAE Systems to work for PricewaterhouseCoopers (PwC), which for me at the time was a huge achievement. He was so annoyed that I left behind a final salary pension. In his mind, the voices in his head, the final salary pension was a really big deal, especially if you worked in a factory. It was a guarantee of a good life when you retired. And he was right. For him it was. But not for me. I wanted to see the world and have different experiences. I would sacrifice the pension for that. I needed to change his voice in my head. I needed to find my voice. I needed to break free from his programming of my thoughts to have my own thoughts.

What did I really want? What new thought did I need to think to get what I wanted? I wanted more than staying in the same job to keep a final salary pension. So I made a decision to leave it behind and move to PwC.

Change your thoughts, change your life

The next part of the book is asking you to listen to yourself and to decide what you really want from your life. To find your true voice. To discover and embed the thoughts that will give you what you want from life. To be brave and find the voice (the thoughts) that can move you to become the best version of you. The you that you really want to become. Not your parents. Not your friends. Not your partner. You! Are you brave enough for that?

At this point, I want to quote Henry Ford, who famously said, 'Whether you think you can or whether you think you can't: you are right.'[11] I also like the quote from Paulo Coelho, from his book, *The Fifth Mountain*. 'If you have a past with which you feel dissatisfied, then forget it, now. Imagine a new story for your life and believe in it. Focus only on the moments when you achieved what you desired, and that strength will help you to get what you want.'[12]

Your past experiences have got you to this point. They have made you who you are today. In this moment. It's time to make what comes next. What you want.

A self-help manual for you

The next few sections have been written to stand alone as a self-help manual. I'm hoping that once you have worked your way through the

---

[11] Foster, 'Whether you think you can ... or whether you think you can't ... you're right', 2013.
[12] Coelho, *The Fifth Mountain*, 2011.

exercises, you will come back to the book and dip in and out of the exercises you found to be the most useful. You may even try them on other people. I have used many of the exercises in my management and leadership roles to bring out the best in the people in my teams. I also still use them in executive and career coaching. That's why I'm confident they'll work for you.

The five-step process

The next part of the book pulls together the best tools and techniques that I have used for over 40 years to become more than my stutter. I have lived and worked in many countries around the world. I've held senior leadership positions for over 20 years and been responsible for the design of people strategies, policies and processes to bring out the best in individuals and teams in large, international organizations. I've coached hundreds of people, built high-performance teams. I've seen the very best and the very worst. I know what works. I've become more than I ever thought I would be as a 17-year-old struggling to say my name and stuck in a job I didn't want to do.

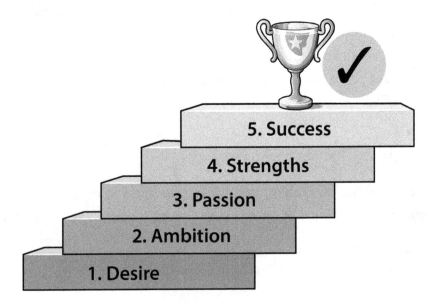

Fig. 1 Five steps to create, live and love the life you really want.

The five-step process will help find your voice, to become more than your stutter and to live the life you really want. Each of the five steps will help you answer the following questions:

- **Step 1:** Desire – How determined are you to become more than your stutter?
- **Step 2:** Ambition – What do you really want from your life?
- **Step 3:** Passion – How will you find the job you love, and love the job you do?
- **Step 4:** Strengths – What are you good at? What is your superpower?
- **Step 5:** Success – How will you get what you want?

In each step you will do a number of exercises, answer questions and be asked to record what you are learning about yourself.

Filling in your Success Summary Sheet

As you work through each exercise, you will capture the output (what you learn about yourself) on a Success Summary Sheet (see Appendices). The Success Summary Sheet will act like your life satellite navigation system (satnav) on a daily basis. You can refer to it before you take your daily actions. You can check it to make sure any decisions you are about to make fit in with your life goals. It's just a really good way to have all you need in one place. You can capture each exercise in the summary or create your own in Word, Excel or in another format that allows you to capture or track your progress and generate a single sheet you can use every day.

What do you want to be known for?

When you think of Joe Biden, Emily Blunt, Tiger Woods, Ed Sheeran, Samuel L. Jackson, Elon Musk, what do you think about them first?

The 46th president of the United States of America, a famous English-born American actress, probably the world's greatest ever golfer, a global musician, a famous American actor, one of the richest men in the world or someone with a stutter?

If you could identify something that you are good at, and become really good at it, could it make your stutter feel less significant in defining who you are? How would you feel if you were known for your talent in sport, running a business, being an actor, an entrepreneur, a fashion designer first, rather than always believing that you are known for your stutter? Is that worth thinking about? As Michelle Obama said in her book *Becoming*, 'I am working towards being the best version of myself, to grow and challenge myself to be the person I want to be.'[13] This book is about helping you take your steps to becoming the best version of you.

Your story questions

- Have you ever read a book that changed your life?
- What were the big lessons?
- How have you used them in your life?

Step 1: Desire

How determined are you to become more than your stutter?

I fundamentally believe that every human being is capable of being more than they are today. But you need to be honest with yourself. Are you really motivated to actually do something about it?

In Step 1, we will discuss:

- Areas of your life you're not happy with
- Your determination to do something different

---

[13] Obama, *Becoming*, 2018.

- Deciding that your stutter will not hold you back
- Writing down your learning in your Success Summary Sheet

In this section you're going to work through a number of exercises to discover why you want to become so much more than your stutter. Not why you should or you could. But what are the real reasons driving you to become so much more than you are today? This will give you the fire in your belly to fight for what you want from your life. That sounds worth knowing. Doesn't it?

Desire is a hunger to make your life better. A determination to put the work in. To learn new things, meet new people, to push yourself outside your comfort zone and to face your fears.

I love the quote from Vinita Kinra, Canadian-born literary artist who said, 'Your success depends on how much fire of the desire you have and how much fuel of passion you feed it.'[14] We need to identify how much fire you have in your belly. But where does that fire of desire come from? If you're serious about making a change, you need to be really honest about how you feel about your life. This can be difficult. But it's the honesty of why you are dissatisfied that will cause you to make a decision to do something different. And give you the energy to make sure you succeed. I had plenty of things in my life I was unhappy with.

I was embarrassed about my job

I was walking back to work from the supermarket at lunchtime (in my early 20s), when a woman stopped my friend and me to answer a few customer survey questions. She asked, 'What do you do for a job?'

I said, 'I'm an engineer.'

My mate laughed and said, 'No, you're not.'

I went red-faced with embarrassment. I was very quiet for the rest of the day. Later on, when I reflected on the incident, I asked myself,

---

[14] Berman, '10 desire quotes to help you build a burning desire for success', 2021.

why did you lie? Secondly, why where you so embarrassed? I had different voices in my head. One voice was saying that *I should be OK with what I was doing. It was a good job. I was being educated. I was skilled in what I did.* The other voice knew that I felt I could do better. I wanted more. It knew I wasn't invested in or proud of what I was doing. My true voice was dissatisfied. But even when I knew that, it caused me a lot of discomfort. Was I arrogant (yikes)? Did I think the job was below me? Not at all. I just wanted more for myself. Answering that customer service question triggered an honest conversation with myself. I wasn't happy!

I dreaded not having enough money

Money in my early 20s was very important. I was married, had a mortgage to pay, we had a young child, with a baby on the way. We always had too much month at the end of the money. I had watched my parents struggle with money, especially in the early '70s. A dispute between the Conservative government and the National Union of Mineworkers caused electricity shortages and the implementation of a three-day working week for many businesses. As a result, my parents struggled to make ends meet and pay the bills. However, as a kid, we always had food on the table. But money was tight. The only chocolate biscuits we ever had were from my uncle, who worked for Crawford's biscuit factory in Liverpool. When he came to our house, he would bring broken chocolate biscuits. Heaven. So the voices in my head were terrified of not having enough money. Finding a way to earn more money was really important. A lack of money was a real driver of unhappiness and worry. I had a real hunger in my belly to earn more money.

Some people are driven to be millionaires or billionaires, and there is nothing wrong with that. I just wanted fewer money worries, and a job I loved and felt proud to say that I did.

I was desperate to inspire others

From an early age I knew I wanted to speak to an audience. I wanted to make people laugh. I had a desire to communicate and explain things. I was good at making complicated subjects easy to understand. If only I could work out when I would speak fluently or when I wouldn't get a block, I could be a great communicator. Or so I thought. At 17, after making a decision to stop all medical treatment to help fix my stutter, I felt an even greater urge to find a way to speak to an audience, the bigger the better. I don't know why. I just felt compelled. As I progressed through my career, I took on bigger projects requiring me to present to bigger audiences. The challenge of my stutter didn't get any easier. But I felt so strongly that my desire to speak in public was my stand against my stutter holding me back. I was more than my stutter and I wouldn't be held back!

I always found starting a presentation traumatic! Normally, when you start a presentation you would say, 'Hello, my name is Paul Gaskin and I'm here today to speak to you about...'; I never did that. I never said my name. If I tried, I would get a block and that would cause me and the audience huge embarrassment. Sometimes, if I got a block at the start of a presentation, it would derail my confidence even if I pushed through it.

I tried all sorts of tricks to get myself going. Maybe a joke I had rehearsed or speaking informally to people in the audience before I started to break the ice. I would often write 'good morning, my name is...' and the subject of the talk on the slide so I didn't have to say it. I then assumed people were reading it as I started the presentation. I would walk around a lot, breathe and then say a word I knew I could say, like 'right', and then launch into the presentation. I found the easiest trick was to get someone else to introduce me. But, alas, there was not always a willing volunteer.

Much later in my career and after a great deal of pain, I found an approach that worked. It went something like this. Regardless of the audience, 10, 100 or 1,000, I would say, 'Right! First I want to cover a health and safety moment.' I would be met by stunned looks around the audience. This is not the topic you should be talking about! I would go on to say:

> I have a stutter. That means, sometimes I get a block. Which means I can't speak. I get stuck! This can last a few seconds. It looks like I'm having a heart attack. I only mention this for your health and safety. Two weeks ago, a bloke in the audience thought he would rescue me from my heart attack. He bustled me to the floor and started to give me mouth-to-mouth resuscitation. Well, I nearly killed him.

Normally people would laugh and that would break the ice for me and the audience. I would then crack on. If I then got stuck, I had already flagged the issue of my stutter. I had a real desire to be a great speaker and didn't want to be stopped by my stutter.

Napoleon Hill, author of *Think and Grow Rich*, one of the 10 bestselling self-help books of all time, said that 'the starting point of all achievement is desire.'[15] I know from my own life and what I wanted that I had to be honest with myself. Why was I unhappy with myself? I had to get the reasons in my head clear.

It's time to be honest with yourself

David Goggins, American ultramarathon runner, ultra-distance cyclist, triathlete, author and retired US Navy seal, describes his life journey from being abused as a child by his father, being poorly educated, having perceived learning difficulties, being overweight and employed as a pest control fumigator with no prospects, and says in many of his interviews, 'You gotta be fu!!@n honest with yourself, you've got to look in the mirror

---

[15] Hill, *Think and Grow Rich*, 2004.

and if you are fat, you have to say man you are fat, if you are lazy you got to be raw with yourself. If you want better you have to take an honest assessment of yourself, if you want more it's down to you.'[16]

Goggins is determined and refreshing. In his inspirational book, *Can't Hurt Me*, he speaks about being a kid with a stutter.[17] Believing that he was stupid, he found it so hard to learn. He was put back a year in school, which reinforced his belief. Goggins was unhappy with who he was, and if he didn't change, what he would become. He took a good hard look at himself. He found desire, a hunger in his belly to become a better version of himself. Today he is a global role model. In talking to himself in honest terms, he set his goals and found his superpower for success. In an interview with Tom Bilyeu, he explains that in his book, he suggests making a list of everything working against you – that there is a lot of power in that list, and you have to accept it before you can fix it.[18]

Your story exercise – it's time to get honest with yourself

I want you to write a list of all the things you are unhappy with in your life and about yourself in your Success Workbook. Use the following list of questions to prompt you.

- What are you unhappy about?
- How do you feel about yourself?
- Your health and fitness?
- Your job or career?
- Your relationships?
- Family?
- Where you live?
- Money?

---

[16] Goggins, Facebook post, n.d.

[17] Goggins, *Can't Hurt Me,* 2020.

[18] Bilyeu, 'Become a savage & live on your own terms! | David Goggins', 2018.

- How you spend your weekends?
- Your character?
- What else are you unhappy with?

Connect with the emotion of your unhappiness. How does it make you feel? This is a conversation with yourself. No one else. If you can't be honest with yourself, Goggins would say, 'You're fu!!k@!d and stuck until you do!' Write as fast as you can (in your Success Workbook), but make sure it's legible. Review the list. Are you sure that's it? What's missing?

How determined are you?

Tom Bilyeu, the American entrepreneur and founder of Impact Theory and co-founder of Quest Nutrition, tells a story of him asking his father-in-law-to-be if he could marry his daughter.[19] He said 'no'. Tom was deeply shocked and embarrassed. His father-in-law-to-be said, 'I have earned enough wealth to ensure my daughter has a great life. I don't see that in you. What do have to offer her?' Tom was honest and said he sulked for a few days. He found it hard to get out of bed. The feeling of self-pity became worse as he chastised himself for not even having the motivation to get out of bed to make a sandwich for his girlfriend, when she came home for lunch. For Tom, it was a matter of personal pride. He made a decision to become wealthy. He didn't know how. He knew he was ambitious to be more than a bum in a bed. Today Tom is a billionaire and an inspiration to many others around the world in helping them to unlock their potential by learning from others.

Your story exercise – test yourself – how strong is your desire to change?

Indicate on the scale of 1 to 10 below, where 10 is a strong desire and hunger to change and 1 is you have no desire to become more than

---

[19] Bilyeu, Instagram post, n.d.

your stutter. Do you have enough raw and honest reasons to change? Time to be honest! Goggins is listening!

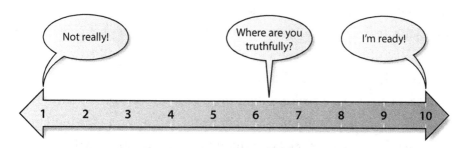

Fig. 2 Honest Self-Assessment: Do you want to become more than your stutter?

Where have you scored yourself? Does that feel right? Do you feel strong emotions when you look at the reasons you have to change and become more than your stutter? Are they strong enough to compel you to take action? From your long list, write down (in your Success Workbook), the really big reasons you are unhappy in as much detail as you can. These are your sources of energy and power. Record your final score (1 to 10) of desire on your Success Summary Sheet.

Make a real decision

Making a real decision is the first critical step to any personal change. Tony Robbins explains the word 'decide' as follows, 'When you make a decision to achieve a goal, you are deciding to cut off any thought of not achieving what you want. You are prepared to do whatever it takes and there is no going back.'[20] The origin of the word 'decide' is from Latin and literally means 'cut off'. This means you tell yourself: I am committed to making this change and this is what it is! You must commit to yourself and override any dissenting voices in your head.

---

[20] Robbins, *Awaken the Giant Within*, 1992.

Your 'eye of the tiger'

'Eye of the Tiger' is a powerful song performed by the American rock band Survivor and is the theme song to *Rocky III*. Having the 'eye of the tiger' means being laser-focused on achieving a singular goal. Being in the 'eye of the tiger' refers to being in a 'kill or be killed' situation. Tigers in the wild tilt their heads to reveal eye-like spots on the backs of their ears just before striking their prey. In *Rocky III*, the boxer, Rocky Balbao, the 'Italian Stallion', is beaten by the young and aspiring James 'Clubber' Lang. Also, Rocky is without his beloved trainer, Mickey, who has died, and Rocky has lost his heart to fight again. Rocky has become a shell of the man he was and he's afraid to fight. Clubber lambasts Rocky into a rematch and Rocky starts training with Apollo Creed, his once boxing arch-rival. The story has a famous iconic scene, where Rocky is training with Apollo on the beach. In the middle of a sprint Rocky stops running. He's done. He's broken. He has lost the 'eye of the tiger'. Rocky doesn't want to push himself. He has lost his reason to fight. Apollo consoles him and says, 'It's over, Rock.'[21]

Rocky has lost his hunger. Lost his desire to fight Clubber. At that moment in time, Rocky didn't have a big enough reason to push himself to the limits required to beat a world-champion boxer more skilled than himself. This is so significant – as an example to us all. At times we all feel beaten or the effort required to reach a goal seems too great. So what will it take? What will it take for you to become determined and change your life? It's down to you!

Later in the film, Rocky, after talking to his wife Adrian, finds a big enough and compelling reason to fight Clubber Lang. He knows that even if he fails to win, he must give it all he has. Whatever the cost to himself. There is no going back! You know how the story ends? He digs deep. Puts his body on the line and wins the fight. Cue the iconic *Rocky* music! Pure desire based on a big enough reason! What's yours?

---

[21] *Rocky III*, 1982.

Your past will define your future unless...

Joe Dispenza, an American neuroscientist, researcher and *New York Times* bestselling author explains how the mind works and how to break patterns of the past to create a new life. I have learned so much from his many interviews on YouTube, where he clearly explains the way in which you have to change what you think to create, live and love the life you want. He describes how we mainly live with our past thoughts, because when you wake up in the morning your brain immediately starts to work on solving problems based on your past experiences. It only knows what it knows. Logically, this means that until you create new thoughts to replace the old and often unhelpful thoughts, you will continue to live the life you don't want. You will keep on repeating what you did yesterday, today and tomorrow. If what you have been doing is making you feel unhappy and unful-filled, logically you will continue to feel that way. It is likely that if you repeat the cycle like a hamster on a wheel, you will either become more unhappy and more unfulfilled or, worse, become apathetic, not care and look for easy methods to dull the pain of unhappiness or to make you feel better, such as alcohol, drugs or dopamine hits from social media.

Dispenza is able to use his research in neuroscience to prove how your brain can create a different life from the one you had yesterday, if you give it a picture and thoughts of the future. You have decided that you want to move away from being dissatisfied with your life and to become more than your stutter. Here is the exciting bit. We are going to imagine and decide what you really want from your life. In the next section, we are going to take the lessons from neuroscience to use the power of your determination and desire to create your new life.

Summary of Step 1

There were four main objectives for Step 1:

1. Detailing a raw assessment of why you are unhappy with you and your life
2. Finding your 'eye of the tiger'
3. Making a real decision to become more than your stutter
4. Capturing your learning in your Success Summary Sheet

Step 2: Ambition

What do you really want from your life?

In my early 20s, after I read *The 4%*, I became very excited and liberated by an exercise which asked me to imagine the things I wanted to achieve year by year for the next five years. I plotted the things I wanted on a simple X–Y axis, so I could see my goals on a single page. I shared the five-year plan with Christine, my wife, to see if she agreed. We both got excited.

Generating that simple picture set my brain in motion. I had never thought about the future in such a tangible way. The voices in my head started to ask, *what if...* I could have a different job, holidays, earn more money, have a nice car and nicer things. I was motivated to be and have more. I just needed to find a way to achieve them. At the time of drawing the simple X–Y graph, I didn't have a clue how I would achieve any of it. I have now learned from smart people how and why it worked. At the time it was an act of faith. A pure desire to be a better me.

In Step 2, we will discuss:

- What you want from your life and what's really important
- Making your new life real in your imagination
- Translating your imagination into reality by writing it out
- Summarizing what you've learned to get focused

In this section we're going to cover a lot of ground. Using a number of exercises, you will brainstorm what you really want from your life. You will use the power of your imagination to create a film in your head of your new life, where you started from and where you end up. You will write a script that describes in detail the achievement of your goals and how you will look and feel when you have all that you want. This is where your fun really starts! If you can imagine it, you can make it real!

The power of your mind

Arnold Schwarzenegger, Austrian-born, American actor, former Mr Universe and 38th governor of California, recalls:

> When I was very young, I visualized myself being and having what it was I wanted. Mentally I never had any doubts about it. The mind is really so incredible. Before I won my first Mr Universe, I walked around the tournament like I owned it. The title was already mine. I had won it so many times in my mind that there was no doubt I would win it. Then, when I moved on to the movies, the same thing. I visualized myself being a successful actor and earning big money. I could feel and taste success. I just knew it would all happen.[22]

Three exercises to awaken your powerful mind

The following three exercises will help you create a detailed description of what you really want from your life and translate your thoughts into reality. I will summarize the exercises before we get into the detail of what I want you to do.

---

[22] Barnes, 'Einstein, visualization and your career', 2021

- Exercise 1: Imagine and write down, without stopping, what you really want from your life, without any inhibitions or constraints.
- Exercise 2: Visualize your priority goals in as much detail as you possibly can, in full colour. Vibrant sound. Strong feelings. Taste and smells.
- Exercise 3: Write down, in as much detail as you can, the priority goals you visualized. Write as though you are producing a script for film director to make a film of your super successful life. How much detail will you need so they get the detail right?

Okay. Now I want you to make sure you are in the right environment to imagine your future. Sit up straight or even stand up. Breathe like you will breathe and feel in the future, when you know you are being how you really want to be. If you're not feeling ready to get excited – do a Goggins. Be honest with yourself and come back to it later. Only do this exercise when you can get excited to imagine the things you really want from your new life. Have some fun!

Exercise 1 – awaken your powerful mind to imagine your new life

This exercise will enable you to create the life you want. Not only what you want but also how you want to feel about you. Please read the following questions before starting to write as fast and as passionately as you can in your Success Workbook.

- What do you really want in your life?
- How will you feel about yourself – what words describe you?
- What are you doing to earn money – what do you love to do?
- Who are your friends – how many do you have?
- Where will you live, what type of house do you have? Get excited
- What does your house look like and where is it?

- What is your health like – how do you look?
- What clothes are you wearing?
- What is your key relationship – do you have a partner?
- How are you with your family – what does it look like, feel like, sound like?
- Where are you holidaying?
- What adventures are you having?
- What else do you have?

Start writing as fast as you can for three minutes. Make sure it's legible. Don't stop; just keep on writing. You should now have a long list. Let's get focused, and prioritize your list.

I want you to divide the list of what you want into three buckets

- Bucket 1: What do you want to achieve within one year?
- Bucket 2: What do you want to achieve within three years?
- Bucket 3: What do you want to achieve in more than three years?

Trust your gut and put the items in the bucket where they feel right. Do some items just stand out as being more important to the core of you? Picking a small number of really important goals will give you more chance of success.

I have completed this exercise hundreds of times with people around the world. There are typical responses from the voices in people's heads. Some worry they are being greedy and asking for too much. Or they worry how will they achieve what's on their list. They worry they will be laughed at by others. Or they won't achieve anything. Others just get really excited and can't believe they haven't done this before. They think it's empowering and can't wait to get started. I have learned through experience that most people, although ambitious, set themselves very stretching yet realistic targets for their lives. Rarely have I seen a ridiculous target. People know what they want. They know deep down inside what's going to satisfy them. So trust the process. Don't overthink it!

If you can imagine it, you can achieve it!

In 1985, Jim Carrey, the famous American actor, when starting out on his career and having not made any films, made an audacious decision. He wrote himself a $10-million cheque for 'acting services rendered', dated it 10 years into the future, and kept it in his wallet. Call it a coincidence, the power of your mind, luck, hard work, talent or a mixture of them all: in November 1995, Carrey found out he was cast in the film *Dumb and Dumber* for – you guessed it — a pay cheque of $10 million.[23]

Visualization is now used as a concrete and proven technique to help people see and achieve their goals. There are many world-class athletes who will state that visualization is a key part of their routine. This includes Michael Phelps, American Olympic swimmer; George St Pierre, one of the greatest UFC fighters of all time; and many others, including Jack Nicklaus, American golfer, and Usain Bolt, Jamaican sprinter – both reputedly the greatest of all time in their field. Many celebrities have also attributed visualization as playing a key part of their success, including Oprah, Will Smith, Arnold Schwarzenegger and Jay-Z; as the latter has said, 'That's how you do it, you have to vision it first.'[24]

It's not only people in sports, films, TV and music who use visualization to imagine their dreams and goals; it has become a much more acceptable and credible approach in business. Businesses spend a great deal of time communicating their vision, mission, strategy and goals with investors, customers, stakeholders and employees in order to share the future direction and purpose of the business. Albert Einstein

---

[23] Bose, 'When Jim Carrey wrote himself a $10 million cheque', 2022.
[24] Jay-Z, *Decoded*, 2010.

once said, 'Imagination is everything. It is the preview of life's coming attractions.'[25] And he was clever. Right?

Exercise 2 – awaken your powerful mind to create a film of your life

Take time to sit in peace and quiet. You're going to use your imagination to make a film of your life inside your head. A film that will show your journey from where you are today to achieving all your goals. It's a story about how you made a decision to break away from the thoughts of your past to create the magnificent life you dreamed about.

Can you imagine where you are when you are celebrating the achievement of all your goals? Is there music playing as you walk towards the celebration event? Who are you meeting and what are you going to do? What can you hear, smell and see? What is your true voice saying to you? Is it a word, a phrase or something else? How excited are you? Visualize all the detail. Imagine you've been asked to make a film of your achievements. A film director has asked to speak to you. They want to make a film of your journey and how you have achieved all your goals. A success film of your life.

Bringing each goal to life

To create a film of your life, we need to give the director and their team plenty of details. Each goal you have achieved will be part of the film. Imagine as much detail as you can to describe the success of each goal. What does it look and sound like when you have achieved that goal? Take the time to imagine the colours, the music that will be playing, the conversations that will be happening. Bring your future to life today. In this moment. Like the script in a film, your imagination has to contain all the details of each scene. This allows the actors, the

---

[25] Einstein and Shaw, *Einstein on Cosmic Religion and Other Opinions and Aphorisms*, 2012.

sound technicians, the prop and costume departments to know what is needed when. The more detail, the better the film.

- What does success look like, sound like, feel like?
- Where are you when you achieve it?
- How do you feel about your achievements?
- What are you saying to yourself?
- Who is sharing your success with you?

Really take the time to imagine the film in your mind. You may need to practise. For some people, pictures in your mind don't work as well as talking to yourself. It doesn't matter. Do whatever works for you, to see you or hear you achieving your goals.

Turning your imagination into the Success Script for your new life

Manifestation is defined as the transition of thought (imagination) into its physical equivalent. It's a term used by many experts, including neuroscientists, to describe writing down your goals and setting in motion the mental process to make them real. You're going to translate all the detail you imagined in the film of your life, in your head, into words. A script. Your Success Script is the description you will use to write down all the details of each life goal you visualized in your Success Workbook. Writing down the details of your film and your goals moves your imagination out of your head and on to paper. More than that. Your brain now has a set of directions you want it to follow. They are no longer just thoughts. It's a plan of action, in words.

Writing it down works!

In 2001, on my many train journeys to and from work in London, I decided to imagine a new life. I had achieved all my original goals using what I had learned from the book *The 4%*. I now worked for PricewaterhouseCoopers (PwC), a prestigious consultancy firm, which

I never thought would be possible. I travelled all over Europe working with global companies to design and deliver big outsourcing projects. Christine and I lived in the house we had imagined all those years before. I earned more money than I believed I could ever earn (even my dad was impressed), and we had started enjoying exotic holidays. But I wanted more. I believed I could be more. I was still restless to find the job which intuitively felt right. I wanted to push myself to be the biggest and best me I could be. I still didn't know what that really meant. I just had a feeling I wasn't done yet!

Here's what happened

I had read a lot of self-help books since reading *The 4%*. Many explained the power of visualization and manifestations. I could see the logic. But to be honest, at first, I was sceptical. Even so, I decided to think bigger and bolder than before. Why not? I visualized what I wanted from my life and created a document of goals for the next 10 years. I saw myself attending the opening ceremony of the Olympic Games in London. At that time, I didn't even know London would bid to hold the Olympic Games. (The London bid for the 2012 games would only be submitted in 2004.) I wanted to live somewhere hot and on a beach. I wrote down very specific details on the location of a gym and a restaurant we would have access to. I even described the specific shape of the beach where I imagined myself running each morning before work. I imagined living and working in countries other than in Europe and earning an income which was much greater than I was earning. Not outrageous, but beyond what I thought a humble factory lad could ever earn. I wanted to push my boundaries to see what I could imagine. An old adage says that if you can imagine it you can achieve it. Arguably one of the most famous manifestations is putting a man on the moon – who would have believed that? John F. Kennedy did!

This sounds unbelievable, but it's true!

In 2010, I moved to live and work in India. While in India, I applied (for myself and family) to attend the opening ceremony of the Olympic Games in London, 2012, and successfully got tickets. How did that happen? It was a global electronic raffle and a completely random process. I applied on the last possible night sitting in the office in Delhi.

I moved to live and work in Hong Kong in 2012 and then to Dubai in 2014. My international career was in motion. In Dubai, we rented an apartment on the famous Palm Jumeriah, which was part of a complex located on the beach. It had a gym on the right-hand side of the apartment complex and a restaurant on the left-hand side. Even more spectacular and unbelievable was the shape of the beach. The restaurant, the gym and the beach were exactly as I had imagined them, all those years before. I can't explain it. But every time I have taken the time to set out my goals in a very considered and detailed way, I have nailed them. Even leaving my last job and starting a different life writing a self-help book that will hopefully inspire others to be more than their stutter. Let's wait and see!

'It happened around five years ago but it's sort of like a mantra. You repeat it to yourself every day. Music is my life. Music is my life. The fame is inside of me. I'm going to make a number one record and the number one hit. And it's not yet, it's a lie. You're saying a lie over and over and over again but then one day, the lie is true,' said Lady Gaga, American singer and actor.[26]

Is it a lie to want to imagine being a better you? Is it not the foundation of the human condition to dream, as many have, to better themselves or their families, towns, countries and the world to be a better place? Greta Thunberg was very young when she set out her vision and passion for a new and environmentally better world. Children dream of playing at Wembley Stadium, the home of English football, or in the

---

[26] Wilcox, 'The law of attraction will never be enough', 2021.

National [American] Football League Superbowl or to win gold at the Olympics.

Jordan B. Peterson, the Canadian clinical psychologist, author and speaker says:

> You must determine where you are going in your life, because you cannot get there unless you move in that direction. Random wandering will not move you forward. It will instead disappoint and frustrate you and make you anxious and unhappy and hard to get along with (and then resentful and worse).[27]

Successful people use the same approach

Athletes and sports professionals imagine (visualize) winning a gold medal or playing for their favourite club. But they neither wait for the universe to present the opportunity nor do they think the universe will make them ready. They know it will take hours of hard work, the right diet, practising over and over again, competing with others for the opportunity to win or play for the team in the final. Manifestation is not a winning lottery ticket, it is the purchase of the belief and visualization of what winning the lottery might give you. Visualization and writing down your goals presents your powerful brain, at the conscious and subconscious level, with a problem to solve. How do we make this happen?

The process of visualization and writing down your goals creates a story for the voices in your head. If you truly believe the story you're telling yourself and you are committed, the new voices in your head will drown out the old ones. The old voices will still try and distract you and tell you that your new story can't be done. They will say you are safer with the old story, your current way of life, your current work,

---

[27] Peterson, Facebook post, 5 November 2019.

friends and lower realistic ambitions. The old voices will find all sorts of reasons why you won't succeed. These are your old voices. Make your goals feel so real and energizing that you push the old voices into the background. You will now start to take action towards achieving your goals. You will wonder why you gave the old voices all that time and space.

Exercise 3 – awaken your powerful mind to translate your film into a script

Your Success Script is a detailed document that you will generate from visualizing your goals in detail. If you were asked to make a film of your life in three years' time, this would be the document you would give to the film director. They would know exactly where you started from and what you have now achieved. Where you live. How you look. What you're saying. This process may take you a couple of hours. It may even take you a couple of days. Revisit it. Close your eyes. Reimagine your goals. Then write them down in as much detail as you can. Some people use pictures they cut out of magazines to supplement their words. Whatever makes your script real to you.

And it works in business, too

I have learned that good tools and techniques apply equally to a work setting as they do to your personal life. You will see practical examples of your Success Summary Sheet and Success Script in many walks of life. A vision or mission statement sets out the high-level goals of a business. Political parties in the UK call their vision and goals for the country a manifesto.

When I first moved into human resources, I worked with an exceptional project director, Terry Standing. Terry was the programme director for the biggest and most critical contract in the BAE division I worked in. It was a failing contract. Behind in production. Failing service trials. Over budget. There was infighting, petty politics, stress and poor morale across the three sites in the division.

Terry brought the top 300 leaders to the headquarters of the division in Stevenage for a three-day workshop. They weren't happy and whined and moaned. They didn't have time for this. They knew what they had to do. Many of the leaders thought the contract was in the toilet and thought Terry wanted to waste precious time giving fancy presentations, which wouldn't change anything. How wrong they were. For the next three days Terry asked only three questions:

1. What were the critical deliverables for the contract and what did success look like?
2. How could we collectively manage risk effectively between design and manufacturing?
3. What specific actions could be taken to accelerate the contract?

What happened next blew my mind

The leaders were divided into tables of 10–15 people and asked to come up with the answers to each question, one at a time. At the start of the three days, there was absolutely no clarity across the 300 leaders of how to consistently answer any of these questions. There were very few tables who had the same view of the critical deliverables. This blew my mind. Terry patiently, without embarrassing people, took us all through what he believed were the key deliverables, the goals (creating the future) for the contract. After a lot of debate and arguing he reached a reasonable consensus of what we had to deliver. He then went on to ask how would we know when we had achieved our goals. Not only would it look like in the end, but what would success look like along the way. So we would all know if we were on or off track.

Each table was set the task to imagine what these milestones would look like, and again a lot of debate and arguing took place until a reasonable consensus was reached. And finally, he asked us to agree to the high-level objectives needed to deliver each milestone. Only three to five things, but we all needed to agree (like in your Success Summary Sheet).

When the leaders on their tables were asked at the end of the three days to play back their understanding of the three objectives, over 80% of people were very clear and 10% were moderately clear. A huge step forward. The leaders were sent away to come up with detailed plans (like in your Success Script) of how each of the three to five objectives would be delivered.

What a life lesson. We left with clear outcomes, clear roles and responsibilities and a collective energy and commitment to get this contract done. It was a huge success and the contract was turned around. The techniques are maybe called different names but, in essence, they are the same. Imagine what needs to be achieved. Visualize what it looks like. Write it down so everyone is clear. Write down the priorities, the top-level objectives or outcomes to be achieved. Write down the detail of what has to be delivered in an initiation document or plan.

I have worked with very clever people all my life. The biggest mistake many clever people make is to assume that the solution to a problem is simple and everyone will know what it is! Really clever people know this is rarely the case. Thank you, Terry!

Summary of Step 2

There were four main objectives of Step 2:

1. Imagine and prioritize what you really want from your life
2. Visualize and bring your future success to life in sounds, smells and feelings in your film
3. Detail all your life goals in your Success Script to make your film real
4. Summarize your life goals on your Success Summary Sheet

Step 3: Passion

How do you find the job you love and love the job you do?

You have now imagined and documented the goals you want to achieve and what your successful life will look and sound like.

In Step 3, we will discuss:

- Finding the job you love to do
- Discovering what you need to always love the job you do
- Finding both is never straightforward
- Recording your personal values in your Success Summary Sheet

In this section you're going to use a number of exercises to understand what you really love to do so you can find the right job. You will learn what motivates you and makes you tick. This knowledge will help you find an organization to work in that shares your view of the world. You will also be able to help your manager understand what you need to perform at your best and be motivated every day. Moreover, you will be equipped with the knowledge to find the career path that aligns with what you want to do with your life. How exciting is that?

Finding the job you love

In my early career, I worked with some really smart guys. Paul Owen was really knowledgeable and a natural with electronics. We worked together to design and build a transfer logic analyzer as part of our Higher National Diploma. Basically, a transfer logic analyzer (TLA) is a piece of electronic kit used to look at the outputs of microelectronic chips. The TLA would capture the digital patterns to test whether the chips worked properly.

During one of the design sessions, Paul casually said, 'This leg of the integrated circuit needs a capacitor to protect it.'

I asked, 'How do you know?'

He shrugged his shoulders and said, 'I don't know. It's just intuitive.' I got out my electronics bible, Horowitz and Hill, *The Art of Electronics*, and found that he was right.

I decided at that moment that I wanted a job which was intuitive. I would just know the right things to do. I wanted a job where I was passionate and enthusiastic. Where I wanted to constantly learn and get better at the subject, because it was fun and interesting. While electronics was fascinating I knew it was not my purpose in life. I couldn't see myself doing it for much longer. I wanted to find a job that I felt had real purpose.

What do you love to do?

Gallup describe themselves as a 'global analytics and advice firm that helps leaders and organizations solve their most pressing problems'. In a recent survey, they identified that 85% of people hated their job.[28] Too many people are stuck in jobs they don't want to do. That's a shocking statistic. I fundamentally believe that if you love what you do, you're going to be so much more productive. You will be happier and learn and grow at a quicker rate than those who don't. Steve Jobs, founder of Apple, had an important message – work is going to fill a large part of your life, and the only way to be truly satisfied is to do what you believe is great work. And the only way to do great work is to love what you do.[29]

You may be saying, that's easy for Steve Jobs to say. I have bills to pay. I do the job I can. Not the job I love. That's a fantasy! You might be right. But what if you're wrong and there's another way? What if I can

---

[28] Clifton, 'The world's broken workplace', 2023.

[29] Stanford News, '"You've got to find what you love," Jobs says', 2005.

help you make the transition to a new and happier job? I have spent a lifetime helping people, including myself (a story which I will share shortly), to find ways to move towards and eventually get the job they want. Some people are fortunate to have a vocation in life, but most people, if we believe Gallup, don't. My daughter, Victoria, spent the first 10 years of her work life working in a variety of corporate jobs. While earning good money, she never felt at home or that they had purpose. She decided to go into teaching. Took a 50% pay cut and has loved her work life ever since!

I've found that when people get stuck or unhappy with their job, they look for another job without understanding what they really want from a job. They don't take the time to understand what they really like to do. 'There comes a time when you ought to start doing what you want. Take a job that you love. You will jump out of bed in the morning. I think you are out of your mind if you keep taking jobs that you don't like because you think it will look good on your resume. Isn't that a little like saving up sex for your old age?' said Warren Buffett.[30]

Your story exercise – what do you love to do?

I want you to think about the jobs you have had in the past and the one you have today. Write down what you specifically like to do. What tasks do you enjoy doing? How do you like to spend your time and why? Equally, write down what you don't like doing. Now this may take you a bit of thinking time. Be as specific as you can. Please use the questions below to stimulate your thinking and write the answers in your Success Workbook.

- How do you love to spend your time in your current job?
- How did you love to spend your time in previous jobs?

[30] Miles Udland, 11 November 2015. 'Warren Buffett thinks working just to beef up your résumé is like "saving up sex for your old age"' *Insider*, www.businessinsider.com/warren-buffett-on-resume-building-2015-11?r=US&IR=T

- What do you like to do at the weekend; how do you spend your time?
- If you could earn enough money by doing what you loved to do – what would that be?
- If you knew you couldn't fail, what sort of work would you do?
- What are you doing when you feel the best about yourself?
- What specifically makes you feel your work has meaning and what is that meaning?
- What are you not doing today that you would love to do?
- What work don't you like doing?
- What is it you don't like about the work?
- What work do you find tedious or boring?
- What work do you find annoying and/or frustrating?

You should now have a few pages of information which can be divided into three lists:

1. The things you love to do (the work, activities, tasks)
2. Maybe you have things you don't mind doing now and then?
3. The list of things you really don't like or want to do!

As a test: if you shared your list of things you love to do with your family, friends and work colleagues, would they agree with you? They will be honest and give you useful insights. These lists may change over time.

What you love to do is unique to you

I worked with an executive assistant whose favourite task was to organize the annual Employee Recognition event. It was a tough project. It took three months to do on top of her already busy job. But she loved the interaction. The feeling employees got from the event and the gratitude they gave her. You may be a restaurant server. Do you like helping people choose from the menu? Making them feel special? Or do you just hate your job and enjoy spending time with animals at the weekend? If you work in a factory or warehouse, do you like learning about and using new equipment? Do you like to be the one that does the hard jobs and solves problems others can't? Do you like to organize others? Or, do you like knowing where all the stock can be found? Do you like analyzing data to solve problems? Do you enjoy creating designs to turn into clothes? Do you like working outdoors with nature?

I eventually found what I loved to do

In my early career, I was involved in electronics, software and systems engineering work. Intellectually, it was interesting. But many of the conversations about circuitry and the detail of programming code or the protocols for the way systems spoke to each other left me cold.

I found the activities I really enjoyed involved talking to people to really understand the problems they were trying to solve. I was fascinated by how a room full of people looked at the same problem in very different ways. I was passionate about getting clarity and a collective understanding of the problem. I found myself naturally getting people to agree to the problem and then what I really liked was achieving a solution as quickly as I could. I found myself to be a natural organizer of people. I didn't have any patience for hierarchy or departmental boundaries that got in the way of the problem I was trying to solve.

I would talk to whomever I needed to get the right people in a room to solve a problem. This sometimes caused me a lot of frustration. As in my early career, I was a bit of a bull in a china shop, and would get very grumpy with people who were obstructive. I would often get a phone call from my boss asking me to stop upsetting the workforce. I just wanted a result! On the other hand, as my career evolved, I started to enjoy the puzzle of getting people to work with me. I remember in my mid-20s, being put in temporary charge of a very smart team of experienced and much older systems engineers who immediately rejected their new younger team leader. Me! But I loved this. How did

I get these guys onside? I had projects to deliver across three locations in the UK, in Lostock, Bristol and Stevenage. There had to be a way to persuade the team to work with me. This fascination with what makes people tick and how you motivate them became a skill I developed.

Increasingly I found myself gravitating towards the leadership of teams, even when it wasn't my job to do so. I just assumed responsibility and made it work. I quickly found that I was a really good number two. The business leader would then just let me get on with running the team, which freed them up to go and do things they wanted to do. I didn't ever want the glory of success. I just wanted to achieve. Finding the job you love is a bit like finding water with a divining rod. You have to trust a force you can't always see. But it's there inside of you. You just need the skills to get the information out. Like an internal satellite navigation system.

How do you find the job you love?

A 2012 article from the *Guardian* suggests that as many as 60% of job vacancies are unadvertised.[31] This was more recently reinforced in an article by Julia Freeland Fisher, who wrote that some estimates suggest that up to 70% of jobs are not advertised.[32] In this article she quotes the CEO of LinkedIn, Jeff Weiner, who has dubbed this the 'network gap'. These are big percentages of jobs that are seemingly not advertised. So if you can clarify what you love to do, and can find someone to help you find what you love to do, you will stand a much better chance of finding the job you really want. In addition, the future world of work is changing. The World Economic Forum suggests that jobs will be very different in 10 years' time, as 50% of jobs will be changed by automation – but only 5% will be lost.[33] Most

[31] I'Anson, 'How to find unadvertised jobs', 2012.
[32] Fisher, 'How to get a job often comes down to one elite personal asset, and many people still don't realize it', 2019.
[33] Van Eerd & Guo, 'Jobs will be very different in 10 years', 2020.

recently, Bruce M. Anderson writes for the LinkedIn Talent Blog that many new jobs will exist by 2030 that look very different from those today.[34] What does all of this mean for you?

Getting clear about what you want to do has never been more important than it is today, as new jobs are being created all the time. Your dream job is out there!

So here is the big lesson. Get really clear about the work that you love to do. A job is a collection of work or tasks. Job titles may or may not describe the work or tasks that need to be done. So by getting really clear about the work you love to do, you can go and find the job that contains more of those elements.

Your story exercise – how do you find the job you will love to do?

You should now have your three lists: the things you love to do, the things you don't mind doing and the things you don't want to do at all. In your current job:

- What percentage of your current job has things you love to do from your list?
- Is that enough for you to love the job you do overall?
- Can you find more of what you love to do in your current job?
- Could you move to a different job in your organization that does more of what you love?

If you cannot find what you love to do in your current organization, then:

- Have you ever seen a job that contains more of the work you love somewhere else?
- Can you estimate the size of the shift you need to make?

---

[34] Anderson, '15 jobs you'll be recruiting for in 2030', 2022.

- If you can't see a job exactly, do you know what industry it will be in?
- Are there people you can ask to help you find a job you love?
- Is starting your own business the answer?

These questions are really important. You need to really understand what you love to do and where that job might exist (as it may or may not be advertised) before changing your current job. In Step 5, we are going to use a problem-solving skill, the Success Action Process, to help you find your new job. Record your thoughts from this exercise in your Success Workbook.

Who would have thought that today you can have a job whispering into our pets' ears to calm and train them, be paid millions as an online influencer, a reality TV star or earn money in online gaming competitions? There are now jobs advertised for big data analysts, digital influencers, creators, cybersecurity directors, wearables developers, specialists in renewable or alternative energy and so many more jobs that were unimaginable 20 years ago.

The world of work is moving so quickly. You may find that what you love to do can earn you money or at least be a key skill that leads to a job that others will pay you to do. Focus on what you want to master and then look for opportunities to develop your knowledge, skills and experience. Find a job you love and open the box to your soul!

How do you love the job you do?

The list you have compiled is how you want to spend your time in work, on the things you love to do. So why is it that people who love their work don't always love or even like the jobs they do? Even those in vocational work like doctors, nurses, actors, musicians can still feel grossly unhappy. They can feel something is missing. Some people can really like what they do. It may not be vocational. But it can be interesting, rewarding, very well paid, include a bonus, good holidays and private healthcare, but they, too, are still unhappy. Some people can go from loving to hating their job. But many people can't quite put their finger on why.

What do you need?

You are unique. What you need to feel happy and love doing in your job is different to anybody else. So how do you pinpoint what you specifically need? When you're loving what you do and enjoying work, you will rarely ask yourself why. You may start to become unhappy in work but not understand what has caused it. How do you find out what's missing when you start to feel unhappy in work? Equally, and I would argue, more importantly, what makes you feel happy in work in the first place?

Your story exercise – let's find out what you need to love the job you do?

If you can get someone else to help you with this exercise it would be really helpful. If not, complete the exercise, and ask someone who really knows you to test if your answers ring true. Repeat the question below over and over again for three minutes. Don't stop until you've exhausted yourself of answers. Keep on repeating the question and write down your answers in your Success Workbook.

- What's important to you about work?
- What's important to you about work?
- What's important to you about work?
- What's important to you about work?

Review your list. Don't change any of the words. The words you have written are very important; they are yours.

Your story exercise – prioritize what you need to love your job

Look at the words or phrases on your list and put them in order of the most important at the top, least important at the bottom.

Your story exercise – test your list to see what's really important

Test your list. When you look at your list, is number two on your list more important than number one? Is number three more important than number two? And so on. Look at your list and order them from top to bottom – does it feel right? Are these the most important things to feel happy and valued in your job? Is anything missing? Typically, what you said first when you started writing your list won't be the most important thing. Don't overthink your priorities. Use your gut feeling.

Using your internal satnav to love the job you do!

Your list is a description of what's most important to you in work. They are your personal values. Your personal values are the conditions or standards that have to be met for you to feel happy in what you are doing. If your conditions or standards are not met, you will automatically start to feel discomfort or unhappy. You don't think about your personal values on a day-to-day basis. But they're like your internal satnav. If you see or hear something you feel you don't like, it's likely to be out of line with your personal values. Your personal values guide you like a satnav to do work and to work with others who have similar personal values to you. Have you ever worked or met with someone and you just get that feeling they're not like you? It's likely that what they think is important about work will not be the same as what you think. It's not a right or wrong thing. It's just different.

What happens when your needs are not being met?

The following is a based on a true story to illustrate the real impact and risk of not understanding someone's personal values.

Sheetal led a large team in a global charity project in Mumbai. She had complete autonomy on how she ran the team, and they were very successful raising funds and delivering projects for the foundation. After a year, the project attracted a great deal of attention from the global headquarters.

When Sheetal prioritized what was important to her about work (her list of personal values) her list looked like this:

- Freedom to act
- Teamwork
- Having fun
- Making a difference
- Leading others
- Values and integrity
- Learning
- Opportunities to progress
- Challenge
- Complexity
- International travel
- Variety
- Holidays
- Good salary and benefits

A new director was appointed above Sheetal to help increase the scale of the project. The new director had a very different style from that of Sheetal's previous director. The new director liked to understand the detail of what was going on and wanted to know exactly what Sheetal and each member of her team were doing on a daily basis.

The new director started to get involved in the day-to-day running of Sheetal's team. At first Sheetal welcomed the new director and looked forward to learning from someone else. But over a period of a few months, she felt suffocated and eventually became very unhappy and resigned. Sheetal felt the new director didn't trust her. The resignation shocked the new director, who absolutely trusted Sheetal; the new director just needed a lot of facts in a new job. Unintentionally, the new director had crossed three of Sheetal's top three personal values. Sheetal didn't feel she had the freedom to act. She didn't feel part of the new director's team and she definitely wasn't having fun. These were unintended consequences caused by the new director.

Your story exercise – why would you leave a job you loved?

Look at your prioritized list of personal values and ask yourself the following question: if you had all the things on your list of personal values, what would cause you to ever leave the job you were in? Record the answer in your Success Workbook. The answer to this question will give you insights into one of your most important personal values. As an example, some people say a loss of trust or ethics, or some might say, I would leave for a bigger job or a family relocation. What's your big reason for leaving a job you love?

Your story exercise – testing your values against your current job?

Let's get really practical and test whether your personal values are being met in your current job. What score would you give each of your personal values, listed from 1 to 10, in your current job (where 10 equals your personal values are being highly met and 1 equals they are not being met at all). For those personal values with lower scores, does this make sense to you? Do you know what's missing from what you need? Do you know how to make the situation better? Alternatively, do you have any high scores and know what the reason is behind that score? What do you need more of?

I have successfully used the values question for over 20 years. In recruitment. Running teams. Assessing people for promotion. Career development. Training people to be managers and executive coaches. People find answering the personal values questions raises their awareness of what they felt, but didn't fully understand why they felt that way. It helps them to understand why they do or don't feel valued in work.

After hundreds of conversations, I have found that money has never been in anyone's top five personal values. This is not a judgement. It's just an interesting observation. Money as a motivator is like a snack. Fulfilling for a moment. But it doesn't sustain you. Most of us want to earn the right amount of money to live the life we want. But the most important thing for most people is to do purposeful work. In a modern world it now has to be both purposeful work and the right amount of money. Ask a Gen Z.

Green light, your gut feeling is right

Matthew McConaughey, in his fabulous book *Greenlights*, uses a traffic-light approach to determine when to proceed with things in his life. 'When things are right,' McConaughey says to himself, 'greenlight – it's OK to move forward.'[35] Do you have the 'green-light feeling' to move forward or is your gut telling you it's and amber (yellow) or red? Pause, breathe, think and reassess.

Your 'green light' is a test of your personal values to any situation. You could say it's an alignment test with your head and heart (some may say soul). It's how you want to be treated and what you need. Next time you get really annoyed with someone, see which of your personal values has been crossed. 'When your values are clear to you, making decisions becomes easier,' said Roy E. Disney, long-time senior executive of the Walt Disney Company and son of Walt Disney.[36]

Imagine you're unhappy in your current job. You're doing what you love. But you don't love what you do because your personal values are not being met. Understanding your personal values will be really helpful when you go for another job. As well as you asking about the work you will be doing you can now ask whether the new work

---

[35] McConaughey, *Greenlights*, 2020.

[36] Colan, 'A lesson from Roy A. Disney on making values-based decisions', 2020.

environment, the personal values of your new boss and those of team will suit you. Are they a match?

Finding a job you love to do, and loving the job you do, can take time. In his book *Transitions*, William Bridges gives great examples of people who take a while to find a job they love and feel at home doing. 'They start in one job, often not knowing what they really want to do. But the job seemed OK at the time. After a while the job became boring or not fulfilling enough.'[37]

When you start to feel it's time to make a change (a transition period), it's really helpful to be alert and listen to yourself to decide what you want from your next job and career. This can take time. People in the wrong jobs may switch jobs in the hope they will find more happiness in the next one. I always say to people, 'Never leave a job before you know what's making you unhappy, or you may jump from one unhappy situation to another to another. After all, everywhere you go, you are there!' Using your personal values will help you find a job you love much more quickly. A good question to ask yourself: is this job and how I spend my time taking me towards more of what I want to do or further away?

In my early 20s, having read the book, *The 4%*, which prompted me to really find the work and a job I loved, I was exploring different types of careers. I went to career counselling sessions. I met people for interviews in many different types of jobs. As a result, I applied for the police. I went to Manchester and sat the police entrance exam. I knew I had performed pretty well. I got to the final part of the assessment, which was a basic health check. The doctor, without looking up, said, 'Name? What is your name?' Shit, shit, shit, always the same hurdle. I was in a long line of people so there was no hiding place. The voice in my head said, *here we go. This is it. Fail time. Here we go. P-P-P... P-P... Paul G-G... G-Gaskin.* The voice in my head said, *not too bad.* I thought nothing of the little stutter until I was told to come out of the

---

[37] Bridges & Bridges, *Transitions*, 2019.

long line of candidates and asked to take a walk down the corridor to another office. 'How long have you had a stammer?' asked the very important-looking police officer in uniform. I asked, 'is it a problem?'

The guy was brilliant. He explained that police work was not as many thought it was. He said that on a daily basis they dealt with many unsavoury characters, who would seize on my stutter and make my life a misery. He was convinced the harassment would be unrelenting. What could I say? He concluded that the job wouldn't be right for me for that reason. He asked the police officer, who had brought me to him, to show me the jobs that supported the police in administration. He wished me good luck. I never thought about working for the police again.

I thought it was worth quickly sharing my career journey to show it's not always straightforward. However, if you keep focused on what you really want you will find a way, even though at times it may not always be clear how you're going to get there.

After my four-year apprenticeship, I had over 10 jobs at BAE. That doesn't include the different projects I worked on. I went from electronics missile technician to standards laboratory technician, software engineering, software team leader, senior systems engineer, computer integrated manufacturing manager, best practice manufacturing team leader, transferring to HR, then HR officer (worst job of my life), HR manager, head of learning and development, deputy head of learning & development MatraBAE (JV). Finally, to head of professional development, BAE virtual university before leaving BAE Systems.

I moved to PwC for just over two years as European Human Resources Outsourcing Programme Lead before being headhunted into Serco where I was employed as HR Director, National Physical Laboratory (NPL), and then progressing to bigger jobs including HR Director Serco Science; HR Director Defence, Science and Technology; HR Director Serco Integrated Transport; HR Director Asia, Middle East, Africa and Australia (AMEAA). My final role was HR Director UK and Europe before I left to set up my own consultancy business and became an author. It took me time and many years of trial and error to work out what I was really good at and what I wanted to do. But each job contained a greater percentage of what I loved to do and what I needed to love the job I did. I was also crystal clear what made me unhappy, and I became much better at assessing a job before I took it.

I had roughly 20 jobs in 40 years. One job every two years. I only really started to feel content with both the work I loved to do, and loving the work I did, when I moved to the National Physical Laboratory, NPL, Serco Group in 2001 (I was 38 years old). That doesn't mean I didn't enjoy work before NPL. It just means I felt more comfortable in myself in the NPL job. The voices in my head and feeling from my heart (my personal values) were much better aligned. I loved being a leader. Doing the right things for the business, in the right way. It didn't mean life became easier. I faced some of my biggest personal and business challenges in Serco. But the struggle was one I wanted.

Summary of Step 3

There were four main objectives of Step 3:

1.   Discover the work you love to do
2.   Gain insights into what you need to love the job you love
3.   Highlight finding both may take time
4.   Record your personal values in your Success Summary Sheet

Step 4: Strengths

What are you already good at? What is your superpower?

We have discovered your life goals, which you have recorded in your Success Script. You have discovered how to find the job you love and to love the job you do. The next step is to understand what you're already good at. Your strengths. Strengths are defined as your natural talents and abilities and any knowledge, skills and experience you may already have. There may be one of your strengths that you could develop and become really good or even excellent at. This will become your superpower and one of the things you are known for. It's also important that as part of this process we understand whether you have any development gaps that need to be closed to achieve your life goals and get the job you love.

In Step 4, we will discuss:

- What you're already good at
- Your potential to have a superpower
- The gaps you may have in your skill set or expertise

Capturing what you have learned to reinforce your strengths

In the books *First, Break All the Rules* and *Now, Discover Your Strengths*, Marcus Buckingham and Curt Coffman make a case from their global research of millions of employees to focus on what people do well in work – their strengths to deliver higher levels of performance rather than their weaknesses. (The old theory was to focus on improving your weakness rather than building on your strengths.) You're going to use all your strengths to achieve your goals.

In this section, we are going to use a number of exercises to build a picture of what you are already good at. Your strengths. I will ask you to review what you are good at and see if you want to develop any of your strengths into deep areas of expertise. Your superpower. I will help you discover what, if any, gaps in your strengths you need to close in order to achieve your goals. It's important to remember that your strengths are going to be very useful to you when you start taking action to achieve your goals in Step 5.

Your story exercise – what are you already good at?

It's no time to be humble. Be bold! Write down (in your Success Workbook) all the things you think you are good at today. It could be working with people, building relationships, making people laugh, influencing, selling. It could be something technical, fixing cars, writing software, creative art design, fashion design, writing. Just think about what you are good at. It could be sport or playing a musical instrument.

What would your family say you were good at? Your friends, work colleagues, even people who may not like you? What would they say? Arguing, listening, solving puzzles? It could be a trait of your personality: hardworking, determined, caring, focused, relaxed, calm, studious, intelligent. Whatever things you believe you are good at, write them down. Are you surprised at the list? Is there a pattern or any groupings?

You should now have a list of things you are already good at. You may also have qualifications or have undertaken some training courses. Have you been the captain of a sports team? Or do you coach teams? When you're at your best, what are you doing? Write it down. Collectively, we will call all the things you are good at your strengths.

Your story exercise – group your strengths

It's worthwhile collecting your strengths together in what seem like sensible groups. This might be the things you know about, skills you have, natural talents, qualifications or experiences. Once you have collected your strengths into sensible groups, can you see any patterns? Are there big groups that show where you have real strength? What surprises you? Are there any areas where you thought you were strong, but you haven't captured much? What's missing? Normally people are surprised by the number of strengths they already have.

Searching for and developing your superpowers

Superman has superpowers. He flies. He's strong. And he can do laser things with his eyes. Other superheroes have different superpowers. The

Hulk transforms into a huge, immensely strong creature. Spider-Man is very strong and has special webs that allow him to travel quickly around the city. Captain America has an indestructible shield and is an expert in martial arts. Each superhero uses their superpower to fight battles. Goodie or a baddie.

Talents

You know people who have special talents. Tiger Woods' father noticed his son was a natural at swinging a golf club from an early age. He spent time developing Tiger's skill. Combined with Tiger's mental discipline and drive to win, he became one of the greatest golfers of all time. Serena and Venus Williams had a similar path. They have natural talent and discipline, and, using a fiercely competitive mindset, became tennis Grand Slam winners. Lewis Hamilton was a natural at go-karting and his potential talent for motor racing was spotted at an early age. With dedication, discipline and that unquestionable competitive mindset, he became a many times Formula 1 motor racing world champion. As with Lewis, Tiger and the Williams sisters, you can see children from a very young age demonstrate natural talent in almost any sport. Football, gymnastics, athletics, rugby, to name a few.

You can also see people in business who are natural entrepreneurs. They are fascinated at an early age with making money and understanding how businesses work. The arts are the same; talented singers, dancers, actors can be spotted at an early age. What were you good at, and/or interested in, when you were younger?

Searching for my superpower

In my transitions from job to job, I was looking for the technical content that I would eventually love to do. I was desperate to become an expert and be known as excellent in something. However, as I spent time in each new role, I found myself asking the same question. Do I want to be great at electronics? Writing software code? Designing manufacturing computer systems? Streamlining the way factories manufacture products? In the end, I realized it was less about the content. It was all about the people and the outcomes they delivered. I had a real passion and belief that everyone can be more than they think they can be. I also fundamentally believe there is a right way to treat people to bring out the best in them. Whether that's creatively or productively. That belief applies to people whatever their differences, at all levels in organizations, across any sector or country.

I also love working in businesses. I enjoy delivering value to customers and understanding the way a business makes money. But more than that, it's the complexity and the wide range of responsibilities a business has to its shareholders, customers, employees, users of the services and economic and regulatory environment that intrigues me. And whatever you do in life, people are at the centre of it, in some shape or form. It's people who make the world work. I was passionate about people. I wanted to develop my superpower to be about getting the best from people and organizations.

At the same time, I read *The 4%* and was getting energized, I attended a week long behavioural development programme for potential managers at BAE. Neil Stringer, a very successful sales and business man, ran the programme. It was a series of group exercises with instant feedback on how you performed. The first task was to agree, with a number of teams, on the additional options (such as an improved sound system, a sunroof, better wheels, to name a few) for a new car, within a specified budget. Well, I won. I argued. I got all my options accepted. Game over. That was easy. In the next task, I got a shock. Although I was made team leader, no one in my team or any other team would work with me.

Time for feedback from the observers. It was brutal and there was nowhere to hide. It was hard to hear. I was loud, aggressive, I didn't listen, I pushed people to my answer. On the second day, over lunch,

Neil started to talk to me. He didn't stop for 20 minutes. On and on and on. OMG. When he stopped I said, 'Is that what I do?' He looked at me. Looked away and started talking to someone else. What a week. I learned so much about personal style, influencing and persuasion, teamwork and myself.

Neil spoke to me at the end of the week and said, 'You're a rough diamond. You just need a bit of polishing.' And walked off. Thanks, Neil, you were right.

I was inspired. He helped me understand I did have a talent to lead teams and get results. But I was a blunt instrument and my style was not sustainable. I set out to learn as much as I could about human interaction, motivation, teamwork and anything I could do to become a very good leader and manager of people. I wanted to be excellent at that. I decided to put an imaginary alarm clock in my head. If I spoke for 30 seconds the alarm would go off. I would stop talking. I did this into my mid-40s. It worked. I learned to really listen and to actually hear what people were saying (I could also hear what they weren't saying).

What are your superpowers?

You may never want to be a world champion in something. But you will have a natural ability to do something. It may be technical or it may be a soft skill. Typically, you love what you do with your natural talent. It won't feel like work.

As you look at your strengths and the work you love to do, do you have any idea what you could be excellent at? If you can find and develop your superpower, you can then apply that to achieving your goals. It may not always be obvious. You may have to discover what your superpower is. You may also have a little cluster of things you are very good at. But over time, one or two things might stand out as the potential superpower.

Your story exercise – do you have any superpowers?

Look at the list of your strengths that you put into groups from the previous exercise. Can you spot any of your strengths that you really love to do and want to get better at? Are there any that you want to define you and who you are? Are there any that if you developed them into a superpower would help you get the job you really wanted? Is there anything missing from your lists? Something that you have always known you want to be great at, but, as yet, you haven't put the time into developing yourself? The next step is to find someone who is already really good at what you want to become great at, and go and find a quick way to get really good, fast. I will help you do this in Step 5.

Do you have any gaps you need to fill?

You now know what your strengths are and what could be a superpower, but do you have any gaps you need to fill?

Your story exercise – do you have any gaps?

When you look at what you want from your life goals within one year, within three years and beyond or to get a job that you love to do, do you have any gaps in your knowledge, skills, qualifications or experience? What's missing? Record your thoughts in your Success Workbook.

You may need help with this question, as you may not know what you need. Certain types of jobs, such as accountants, doctors, police officers, business consultants and software engineers, require specific qualifications or a track record of experience. Or require working in other countries or sectors. There are no insurmountable barriers. However, it's worth checking what is required, so you know what you need to do. When I worked at BAE Systems, most senior technical and engineering roles required a relevant degree-level qualification to be promoted. I, therefore, did a degree in mathematics, software and systems with the Open University (OU) (online learning). However, there are many roles that do not require formal qualifications, so don't be put off!

In a competitive world you need to be very good at whatever you do to be successful. As Tom Bilyeu, American billionaire entrepreneur, author and co-founder of Impact Theory says, 'The key to becoming successful is to work so ridiculously hard at acquiring skills that when people see how good you are they just assume you're naturally talented.'[38]

Even people who are hugely talented practise their skills to become great at their craft. Whether that's in sport, business, music, art or whatever they are passionate about. Although to be fair, everyone requires a bit of luck along the way. My aim is to focus on what you are good at and to develop what you feel you could be great at in order to maximize your belief in yourself and minimize and shrink the impact of your stutter. T. Harv Eker, Canadian author and motivational speaker, summarized the point brilliantly when he said, 'Success is a learnable skill. You can learn to succeed at anything.'[39]

Summary of Step 4

There were four main objectives of Step 4:

1. Understand what you're already good at – your strengths
2. Identify and develop your superpower
3. Understand any gaps and what more you need to learn
4. Summarize and fill in your Success Summary Sheet

Step 5: Success

How will you get what you want?

At this point you have a Success Script that describes what a successful life looks like for you. You understand the work you love to do and what you need to love doing that work. You understand the strengths

---

[38] Hamre, 'Tom Bilyeu's most inspirational advice on how to achieve greatness', 2021.
[39] Eker, *Secrets of the Millionaire Mind*, 2005.

you currently have, any potential superpowers, and what else you may need to learn to achieve your ambitions.

In this section you will use exercises to implement a proven set of five skills to convert your goals into reality. When you have implemented Step 5, you will start to see, touch, feel and hear what you imagined as your new life, as it morphs into your day-to-day life. Invest in learning the five new skills and you are choosing to invest in you!

You are the architect of your life

Imagine you're working with an architect to design the house of your dreams. You visualize your house and work with the architect to translate the pictures in your head into a three-dimensional design. You can now see what the house looks like inside and out. They have brilliantly brought your thoughts to life. You can see the position of the house on the plot of land you have bought. You can see the driveway and how it curves a little before going through wrought-iron gates onto the road. You can see the shape of the roof and the number of windows and doors. You can see where the garage is located. The shape of the garden and boundaries. You have an overview of the house without the detail. The three-dimensional image is similar to your Success Summary Sheet, which is a summary of your new life without the detail. When you close your eyes, you can imagine all the things on your Success Summary Sheet like it's a three-dimensional image.

You need a builder

You're now sitting with the architect to generate a detailed plan and a list of materials (all the stuff you need to build the house). You work together to design each room. Paint. Fittings. Toilets. Showers. Tiles. Internal doors. Window blinds. Light fittings. And, finally, the kitchen in all its glory. The more detail you can imagine, the more detail the architect can give the builder, the better the chance they will deliver the exact house you want.

Working with the architect is the same as you imagining, in detail, your life goals described in your Success Script. Each of your goals is imagined like a room in the house. You have written and captured what each goal will look like, when you have successfully achieved them. Your Success Script describes the richness in words of what you will see; the sounds, smells and feel that let you know you are living your new life. You can see where you will be and what people will say to you when you know, *I've done it!*

The architect selects a builder they know and trust to build your house. The builder is known to have built many magnificent houses before. They have all the tools and techniques they need to turn the three-dimensional image, and the detailed drawings, plans and list of materials, into a real house.

Five practical skills to make your new life real!

You are the architect and builder of your new life. You have done all the design work. You have detailed plans. The question is, how will you get what you want? How do you move from words on a page (your Success Summary Sheet and your Success Script) to your new daily reality?

There is only one way. You need to take action. Taking action everyday will move you steadily towards the life you really want. To help you take the right actions and make them stick we are going to use five new skills. These new skills are proven to work and are very practical. Like the builder we described earlier who was building your house, laying bricks needs practice. The five skills we will use will also need a bit of practice. But their use every day will bring you brilliant results.

In Step 5, we're going to use your five new skills to deliver your life goals:

- Skill 1: Success Action Process – Translating your thoughts into actions
- Skill 2: Mental Metal – Developing your mental strength
- Skill 3: Time-shifting – Making time to create your new life
- Skill 4: Success Workbook – Reflecting on what does and doesn't work
- Skill 5: Brilliant Networking – Finding role models to get you faster results

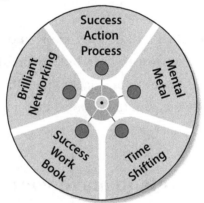

Fig. 3 Five new skills to deliver your life goals

Skill 1: Success Action Process – translating your thoughts into actions

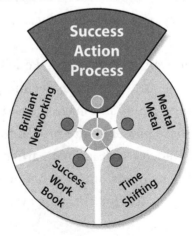

Fig. 3a Skill 1: Success Action Process

Your story exercise – translating your thoughts into action

Look at your Success Summary Sheet. Pick the first life goal you feel most compelled to achieve. Immerse yourself in the detail of that goal in your Success Script. Remind yourself what it will look like and feel like when you have made this goal a reality and you have achieved your outcome. We're now going to achieve your goals brick by brick. Or action by action. We will start by using a very simple process to take daily action towards the achievement of your goals.

Success Action Process

1. Write down one of your goals (the outcome you want)
2. Take one action towards achieving that goal (possibilities, choice, action)
3. Review, learn and move on (assess, learn and adapt)

Surely it can't be that simple? Yes, it can. If you repeat the process each day, every action you complete will build momentum and drive your life forward.

Your story exercise – practise with the Success Action Process

1. Write down one of your goals: this is the outcome you want to achieve
2. Take one action towards achieving that goal: select the action that moves you forward
3. Review, learn and move on. What did or didn't work? What did you learn or need to adjust?

What did you notice when you did this? Was your action real and practical? Don't worry if it's not clear yet. We're going to do some worked examples to help you practise. Tony Robbins says, ' Never leave the scene of a decision without taking action.'[40] Action really does

---

[40] Robbins, *Awaken the Giant Within*, 1992.

mean that what are you going to do is practical and tangible. A simple action could be making a phone call. Doing research on the internet to learn something new. Reading the chapter of a self-help book. Eating one less piece of toast. Going for a 10-minute run. It could be finding someone new to talk to who could help you. But make the phone call. Find a gym. Set your alarm earlier to create an extra 30 minutes a day. Buy a book that gives you more knowledge about what you love to do. You could create a simple plan in your Success Workbook about how you will get your new job or look at options to start a new qualification or training course. Practical. Practical. Practical.

The Success Action Process might feel awkward at first. You're asking the voices in your head to do something different. Your current routines are strong and powerful. They don't want you to do new things. The old voices in your head think, 'It's much safer to keep on doing what we've always done.' Doing the same things over and over again are called habits. Imagine you haven't got a mobile phone, because the old voices in your head said that 'landlines are much better'. Is that stupid? Yes, it is! But it's exactly the same. New thoughts, new actions. New habits. Move forward. Just do it!

A bit more explanation of the Success Action Process

Imagine your goal is to get a job you love more than the one you're doing today. You have identified the tasks you love to do and what you need to love the job you do. You're clear about the type of work. But maybe not what type of job. This is something you need to find. You have some clues. You've already written a very detailed description of the job you love in your Success Script.

In the worked example, when you're in the job you love:

- You are designing new clothes for the teen market
- You are working in London
- The offices are funky and a bit wacky

- There is a buzzy atmosphere and lots of creativity
- The team are young like you and promotions are based on talent
- There is the potential for international travel
- You want to be trained to use the latest technology in design

Today you work as a trainee accountant in one of the big four consultancies. You're well paid and work long hours. Let's find your new job using the Success Action Process.

Success Action Process: a worked example

- Write down your goals. My outcome is to work in a job I love, in the fashion industry. Timescale, within three years. I want to make fashion designs that are funky and fun to wear. My target is the 15- to 19-year-old teen market.
- Take one action towards achieving that goal. First of all, let's understand what possible options you have. Research the internet for fashion recruitment consultancies. Could you ring a fashion house and ask for a chat? Have you started to create any of your own designs to see if it's something you would really like to do? Do any of your friends have any contacts in the fashion industry? Does the accountancy firm you work for have any links with a fashion house? Are there any fashion shows that you can get an invite or go to, so you can meet people from the industry?
- Secondly, which possible option should you choose? Your choice will be based on your gut feeling and common sense. Maybe you talk to a trusted friend. But don't overthink it. The important thing is to choose an option. Susan Jeffers, in her book, *Feel the Fear and Do it Anyway*, says 'there is no right and wrong answers, only learning. Make the decision and learn.'
- Thirdly, take the action. Do it. Make the call. Whatever you decide. Do it that day.

Finally, when you have completed the action, assess whether the action moved you towards finding the job you want. Did it work? If not, why not? What did you learn by taking that specific action? From what you learned, will you do something differently next time? Your momentum will be built by taking lots of actions, quickly. Learning what works and moving on to the next action. Failure is success. It tells you to try something else.

Put into practice: I need to change jobs

I used the Success Action Process when I decided to leave PwC, a company I was very proud to work for. But I wanted to find a job that had more alignment to my personal values and the type of work I ultimately wanted to do.

My biggest job at PwC was to lead a project to simplify, standardize and outsource HR transactional services of 17 European countries for Nortel Networks, a global telecommunications company. The service would be delivered from a PwC multilingual call centre in London that we would build, with service levels and a mutually beneficial commercial agreement. The project was the most complex part of a $635 million global deal to help Nortel deal with its unprecedented growth. I definitely had imposter syndrome. I had not done anything like this before. No one in PwC had.

There were a number of significant challenges to the project:

- Nortel managing directors and human resource directors didn't want HR outsourced
- Each country wanted the new service centre in their country
- Policies, processes and employment law were different in every country
- Timescales and the budget were impossibly tight

After huge self-doubt about my ability to deliver the project, I looked at myself in the mirror and challenged myself to have a go. I did.

I used my strengths in building relationships and understanding what motivated people. I persuaded each of the Nortel national managing directors and human resource directors that we could successfully outsource and improve the service they were getting locally. We would do this more cost effectively, and we would use the new service to outsource more of their work over time. Most importantly to Nortel, I was able to demonstrate that we could satisfy the legal and data requirements of each country and the simplified processes would deliver over 80% standardization. This would reduce service delivery risk, improve quality and provide a foundation to take on more work as they grew.

The pressure to deliver to the project budget and ever-tightening deadlines became overwhelming. I wasn't seeing my family. I was working more than 12 hours a day, including working long weekends. I was travelling to a different country in Europe every other day and becoming exhausted. I was running out of ideas of how to make the project go faster and the complexity was increasing. PwC had given me a budget based on what we were initially charging Nortel. But I needed more resources to hit the deadlines. I could see there were people in the PwC office who were not working for clients, but the partners told me the budget would not allow me to have more resources.

One Friday night I arrived home at 11:00 p.m. My family were in bed. I had a cup of tea. Set the alarm for 5:00 a.m. I was meeting the lawyers on Monday. The legal schedules for the commercial deal had to be completed by then. It was 5:45 a.m. and I was on my second cup of coffee and working through a legal document when my young son appeared at the door, wiping his sleepy eyes, but so happy to see his dad. 'Daddy, you're home?' 'Son,' I said, 'can you please go back to bed for an hour?' I still remember the disappointment on his face. I felt awful and such a failure. I was putting work before my family. I was putting work before everything. I didn't have a life outside of work. And I wasn't enjoying what I was doing.

I took a long, hard look at myself. It wasn't easy. I could blame the PwC partners for not giving me more resources. I could blame the complexity of the project. My own team for not working hard enough. Nortel for being so demanding. Myself for not being good enough. An old and easy target. It was clear the project was having a negative impact on me and my family. And I had got myself stuck in a thinking rut. Work harder. Work more hours. Willpower will get me over the line. It was an old mantra and it wasn't working.

On Monday morning I went to see the PwC partner responsible for the project. I said, 'I want the people I need to deliver Nortel. I will deliver the project successfully. Then I will leave.' I did and I did. My son caused me to change the voice in my head. He gave me the desire to change my thinking and my actions. I didn't blame anyone else for my situation. I made a real decision. The decision caused my mind to shift and look at other possibilities. Not only did I get more resources. It opened my mind to deliver the project in a different way. I made different choices. Remarkably, within two weeks I found myself with an abundance of time. I took action and I achieved the right outcome for everyone. Including the budget. It was a real negative that became a positive. I learned so much about myself. I love the little adage, 'If it's going to be, it's down to me.'

Your story exercise – when did you learn the most about you?

In your Success Workbook please answer the question, have you ever felt you have failed hugely? But on reflection, have you learned the most?

- What was the situation?
- What happened?
- What did you learn about yourself?

Working for PwC had opened my mind to so many possibilities and opportunities. I had successfully worked with global leaders and multifunctional, multinational teams in Nortel and PwC to deliver a very successful, complex and profitable project. Not only that, it was a completely new field of working to me and those I had led. I had built a brilliant team who were highly motivated and succeeded in unbelievable circumstances. I now knew, for certain, I was capable of more.

How I used the Success Action Process

I felt I wanted more; however, the job couldn't be the same. But what did I want? I needed a really big personal shake up. I needed to find greater levels of clarity to understand the work that I really wanted and needed to do. I used the Success Action Process to help me. It was time to reset my life goals. I needed to get myself into the right state of mind. I felt I needed to a take a number of short-term actions.

- **What was my goal?** To get myself into the right state of mind to reset my life goals and create a better life for myself and my family.
- **Possibilities, Choice, Action** – What options did I have? Find someone to help me? Buy a new book? Go and speak to an executive coach? Find a course I could go on? I needed a catalyst to create space in my head. Then I saw an advert for a Tony Robbins Awaken the Giant Within event in Cardiff. I immediately applied and paid for the four-day programme, without really reading what it entailed. It just felt right.
- **Assess, learn and adapt** – I knew I needed something different. I now wondered if I could reclaim the money I had paid for the four days from PwC or if I would need to pay out of my own pocket.

I attended the Awaken the Giant Within event and fully immersed myself, including doing a fire walk. As a result of the four days, I made new decisions that allowed me to get my head in the right place. I became much clearer.

What were my revised short-term goal(s)?

To successfully complete the Nortel project and get another job. My new thoughts were to find a job that felt more aligned to who I was. What I needed and what I loved to do. To get my head in the right place. To revisit and write a new set of compelling life goals. To get better balance and start to enjoy my life, rather than just working.

Action(s)

I made a decision at the event to give up alcohol, caffeine and meat for at least a year. Decided to set fitness goals and complete the Great North Run in September. Decided to restart my journal and design a life I really wanted to have that I could enjoy and be proud of. I shared in Step 2 that I had written a 10-year plan of goals. The Tony Robbins event was the catalyst I used to change my thinking. I also decided to set time aside each day and at the end of the week to review my actions and progress. I wasn't completely clear where I was going but I knew I had to take action to make me think in a different way. I had to create a plan of things to do that would break my current habits.

Assess, learn and adjust

I learned that sometimes to make a big change you need to take yourself out of your current environment, work and home. I needed to completely immerse myself with new and different inputs to really shake my thinking. The complete immersion meant I had no room to keep going round and round the same problems in the same way. Tony Robbins and his team caused me to interrupt my thinking. I now had a set of actions to move forward.

Within six months I had been headhunted by Serco. Lost weight. Got fit. And got myself a prioritized set of goals for the next five years. In the next section we will explore one of the unforeseen problems of changing yourself. Other people don't often like it.

Skill 2: Mental Metal – developing your mental strength

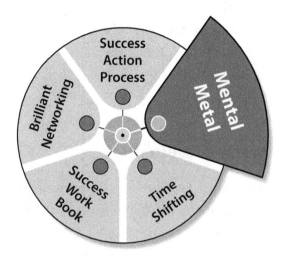

Fig. 3b Skill 2: Mental Metal

This may sound a little dramatic, but you will need to fight for yourself and what you want. If you don't, you will do what others want you to do; that's just life. George Patton said, 'Better to fight for something than to live for nothing'.[41] Why can't that fight be for you, to become more than your stutter? You are either shaping your life, or others are shaping it for you.

Who do you think you are?

The truth about most people – and you know this to be true – is that, for all their moaning, they're happy in life where they are. But they're also happy that you are with them in their world. Doing what they're doing. Having their conversations. Being part of their routines. Because that's their safe space. When you start on your journey to become more than your stutter, you may be surprised by the reaction of your family, your friends and work colleagues. Changing your thinking and your habits

---

[41] Brighton, *Patton, Montgomery, Rommel*, 2010.

can be perceived by others as you questioning their lives. I know it sounds bizarre, but other people can think, 'Who do they think they are doing a qualification, taking extra courses, moving from our town. Are we not good enough anymore?' I only say this to prepare you. People have put you in a box. A box they know and understand. You now want to break out of your box, but also their box. That won't be comfortable for everyone.

What's the link with stuttering?

Arnold Schwarzenegger became the governor of California after he had become a successful actor and businessperson. He became a successful actor as a result of winning Mr Universe. He became Mr Universe after deciding to become more than he was at the time by breaking muscle to become physically and literally a bigger and better version of himself. Your personal growth will result in you breaking new mental muscles. You will create new and bigger thoughts finding out what you want to do, making that work, learning, failing, learning, succeeding. The achievement of each life goal will increase your confidence and choices in life. You may still live with your stutter. Arnold has not completely lost his Austrian accent. But does he care? You will care less about your stutter as you become more. Does Arnold worry he is no longer Mr Universe? I doubt it. He has grown beyond that stage of his life and become so much more.

Your story question: who has already opposed your change?

Have you ever tried to make a change and felt held back by others?

- What was the change?
- Who tried to hold you back? Alternatively, who tried to help you?
- What did you do?
- What clues does that give you about you and your ambition?

How long does it take to make a change?

There are different opinions. Tony Robbins says that 'you can change what you think in a heartbeat.'[42] I agree. You can. But to keep on doing new things, even when you have decided, also takes discipline and time. According to a study published in the *European Journal of Social Psychology*, it takes between 18 and 254 days to form a new habit.[43] On average they say it takes 66 days before the habit becomes automatic. I have found that, realistically, it takes a good 10 to 20 days to change and maintain a new habit. But it can be achieved.

Think of people you know who go on a diet or go to the gym to get fit. Some people go to the gym for two weeks. Mainly in January. Before they give up. Some may last three months. Others will go longer. But if they keep going to the gym for longer, they are likely to sustain the change of their fitness habits as a way of life. My son was nearly 95 kg at the age of 17. He saw himself on a video while in a school production of *Les Miserables*. Three months later he had dropped nearly 19 kg and has maintained a disciplined weight since then. He is now 35. An instant decision. But daily discipline and years of working to maintain his fitness.

Tough decisions are often made by you alone

It is inevitable that a small number of decisions on the journey to achieve your goals will be life-changing. Those decisions will really challenge and push you outside your comfort zone. They may even make you frightened. A decision that you know, if you make it and take action, means there is no going back to the old you.

These decisions are often about making a stand for yourself in the face of huge challenge and adversity. It's worth keeping your internal antenna tuned to hear these moments. The thing is, only you ever

---

[42] Smulders, '100 lessons from Tony Robbins' "Unleash the Power Within 2018"', 2022.

[43] Lally et al., 'How are habits formed', 2010.

really know what they are. Because only you know who you want to be. And only you will live with the voice in your head. This can be a lonely, but important, place to be. Don't shy away from those big decisions. Is it better to regret a decision you don't make, or regret a life you could have had? If you're not feeling resistance to change, either from yourself or others, you're not pushing yourself hard enough.

Building momentum, one action at a time

If you do one action a day using the Success Action Process, you will have achieved 365 actions in a year. Over 1,000 in three years. The biggest challenge is doing your actions when you don't feel like it. It's having the personal discipline, knowing that one action every day will deliver your life goals over time. A builder knows they have to lay a specific number of bricks every day if they are to build your dream house on time. It's the same principle. You're the builder of your life. Action by action. A builder is also very clear how much time they need to build the house. They can't cut corners, or they will build a sub-quality house. You need dedicated time each day to deliver your life goals.

Skill 3: Time-shifting – making time to create your new life

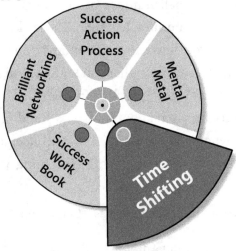

Fig. 3c Skill 3: Time-shifting

I don't have time

The biggest barrier I hear to personal development is always, 'I don't have time!'. It's the same excuse in every country I have worked. It's the same about work. The mantra, 'I can't do a new project. I don't have time. I can't do more. I don't have time!'. We all have 24 hours a day. It's a choice how you use them. I have personally suffered from the same voice in my head. *I don't have time.* You do have time. But something else has to shift. Life is a trade-off. A trade-off, of your time and energy. I estimate that you will need an hour a day to achieve your goals. That's 4% of your day. You can start with less time and build up. But you don't get the life you want for free.

I completed a four-year Open University Degree while working a full-time job. I also worked overtime and a part-time job at the weekends to pay the mortgage. We had two children under the age of eight and I still kept up some level of sport. I wanted more for me and my family. There will always be sacrifices in the short term to build the life you want in the longer term. The truth. You can't have it all. At the same time. But you can have it all. In time.

Your story exercise – how do you spend your time?

For 14 days keep a detailed diary and write down what you do with your time. Be as granular as you can. There is no judgement here. It is what it is. We all have different roles and commitments. An example could be:

Day 1, Monday
6:30 a.m. – alarm goes off – press snooze
6:40 a.m. – check phone, bathroom – toilet, shower, teeth, get dressed
7:00 a.m. – have breakfast, wake kids, pack bag, find car keys
7:15 a.m. – commute to work
8:00 a.m. – start work
12:30 p.m. – lunch

1:00 p.m. – continue working

6:00 p.m. – drive home

7:00 p.m. – get home, put stuff away, help make tea

7:30 p.m. – bathe kids and get them to bed

9:30 p.m. – watch TV

11:30 p.m. – bed

You should have a comprehensive list of activities for each day, including how you spend your time in work.

Your story exercise – find one hour a day to become more than your stutter

Look at how you have spent every 30 minutes of the last 14 days. How much of your time is devoted to achieving your goals? How much time do you spend watching TV (the average person spends up to three hours per day). Can you find 4% in your day (60 minutes) to work on your dreams?

Your normal routine

When you look at your last 14 days, do you see any patterns? You may be doing the same things at the same time every day. Having a routine in your daily life is critical. On a practical level you need routine just to get through the day and to get things done! However, most people drift into their routines. When you examine your days, you may be surprised how repetitive they are and where you spend your time. Be honest with yourself. You can see opportunities to shift or stop doing some things, can't you?

The things you do over and over again are your routine (habits). Routines are the things we do consistently. Often without thinking. They're in your subconscious. Like breathing. We don't need to think about them. Each day you get up when the alarm goes off and your routine automatically clicks into gear. Get up, brush your teeth, shower, get dressed, breakfast, get in the car, go to work.

However, when your circumstances change, you get a new partner, you have children, you start a new job, the old pattern is interrupted and you transition to a new pattern. You may feel discombobulated for a while and then you settle into a new routine and new pattern of how you run your life. Therefore, routines are not fixed in stone. You can choose to vary them. And forces outside your control can also vary them for you.

Shifting your routine

To achieve the life you want, you need to change your old routines and create new ones. Or at least interrupt the old routine and insert new tasks. This requires a change in thinking and discipline. Thinking is the voice in your head that says, 'I should do something.' Discipline is the consistent action you take to improve yourself, whether you feel like it or not.

Let's use the Success Action Process to help you find an hour a day

Write down one of your goals. To create one hour every day to create my new life and take at least one action to move me in the right direction.

Action(s). Take one action towards achieving that goal – document how I spend each 30 minutes every day for 14 days. Look for possibilities to remove, shift, combine or not do certain tasks to create the hour a day. I have decided to set the alarm clock for 5:45 a.m. Monday to Friday and 6:45 a.m. on Saturday and Sunday to create an hour in my day, for me.

Assess, learn and adjust. What did or didn't work? What did I learn? Need to adjust? I will need to assess if getting up earlier is helping me or not. I will review my decision in four weeks to see if it's working.

Your story question: when is your hour?

After working through the exercise, have you decided and committed to a time in the day to spend an hour on you? When is it? Write it down in your Success Workbook.

Where could you get more time from?

The 2020 Ofcom report in the UK found we spent more time online than previously.[44] An average of 3 hours 37 minutes a day on smartphones, tablets and computers (9 minutes more than in 2019). An average of 1 hour 21 minutes a day watching online services such as Netflix and BBC iPlayer on TV (24 minutes more than in 2019). Most people in life are happy where they are. They will moan and say they want more. But most are not prepared to think and act differently. In three years' time, they will still be online and watching TV. What are you going to be doing?

You have now found an hour a day. You could really improve how productive you are by making the hour you have found the first hour of your day. This may take a little time, but the evidence from many of the most successful people in business is that the first hour sets you on course to be super focused and productive.

It really is common sense when you think about it. Mobile phones, checking your emails or social media, turning on the TV or radio are all distractions about other people and what they want from you. The first hour of your day could be all about you creating your future!

I love the Mel Robbins quote, 'Don't miss your life because you are too busy scrolling through somebody else's.'[45] Robin S. Sharma has a 20:20:20 methodology to own the first hour of his day: 20 minutes for exercise, 20 minutes for gratitude and 20 minutes to learn something new each day.[46]

---

[44] Ofcom, 'Online nation', 2020.

[45] Robbins, Twitter post, 2017.

[46] Drake, 'VALLEY tries it: Robin Sharma's 20/20/20 method of the 5 a.m. club', 2022.

Own the day or it owns you!

Finding your own way to spend the first hour will be important. I always made sure I had my weekly and daily objectives front of mind as well as some physical exercise. It's the daily discipline that will prove to be most valuable to you. You will find what works for you. But get focused. Would you get in your car not knowing where you are going or let someone else determine your travel destination? No. Why would you do the same with your day? Own the day or it owns you. You know this is true!

Your story exercise – how will you spend the first hour of your day?

Use the Success Action Process to work out the best way for you to start your day. What things do you want to do that put you in the best state of mind to deliver your life goals? This is a lifestyle change. A change of habit. A new discipline. Apply the same process to your job and see what happens.

Skill 4: A Success Workbook – reflecting on what does and doesn't work

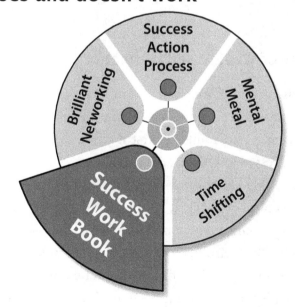

Fig. 3d Skill 4: Success Workbook

Get it out of your head

In a complex and ever-changing world, which at times can be over-whelming, a journal can be a quiet companion. I used to leave my journal at the side of my bed. Oftentimes, when I worked on a big project, I would wake in the early hours of the morning. My head buzzing. I would write down my thoughts in my journal and go back to sleep. A place to record your deepest thoughts and insecurities. Get them out of your head and down on paper. This act of transfer from mind to paper is cathartic. It's a great skill to help you make sense of your thoughts.

Use your Success Workbook on a daily basis

Engineers always record what they do in a log book. It's an age-old tradition. I was the same. You keep track of what works and what doesn't. But also, you record good ideas. Entrepreneurs like Richard Branson do the same. It's a great way to capture new business ideas. I think it's a really good daily discipline to help you in the achievement of your goals.

The power of weekly self-reflection

Taking one hour out of your week to reflect is also really important. Throughout my career I have made time to reflect on my week in work and in my personal life; at first it was at least an hour a week. Then as I progressed into bigger roles, I made sure I dedicated more to reflection time. My executive assistant used to tell people, 'Paul can't be contacted unless it's urgent, it's Friday afternoon. Paul's thinking time.' If I was working on a complex problem or a big project, Friday afternoon would be consolidation, creation and thinking time. When I moved into senior leadership roles, it would be thinking of the future, developing strategy and planning what next. But first, always a time for reflection. On Saturday morning I would often get up early and write down what I thought about the week that had just gone. What had gone well and not so well? Most importantly, what could I learn and do differently?

Effort does not always deliver success

There is a lovely story of the army using machetes to hack through the Amazon jungle. A young corporal climbs up a tree and shouts, 'Sergeant, we're going the wrong way!'. The sergeant responds with vigour and authority, 'Don't bother me now, son, we've just started to make progress.' I have learned to fight against the corporate machine and myself to ensure that I take time to pause, reflect and assess, is what I am doing right? You don't always get that chance. But more often than not, if you don't you will lose yourself.

Learning from the experiences you have had in the week will require some quiet time and reflection. It is therefore important that you choose a time and a place when you will be on your own, away from any distractions. I found that reflecting first and then sometimes checking or testing my thoughts with someone else I trusted was always very productive to my progress.

Your story exercise – optimizing your weekly self-reflection time?

Decide when will take the time out of your week to reflect on the week's events? Put time in your diary now and write down your decision in your Success Workbook.

Skill 5. Brilliant Networking – finding role models gets you faster results

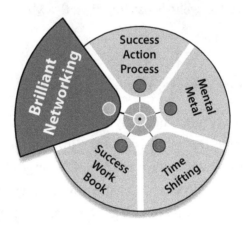

Fig. 3e Skill 5: Brilliant Networking

One of the best pieces of advice I was given as a young, ambitious engineer was to find the person doing the job I wanted to do next. This was brilliant advice. Denis Waitley said it best, 'The primary success factor is knowing how to learn from others, and rely on yourself.'[47]

Not only did I find a role model for my next job, I started to look at the traits of people I wanted to be like or not to be like. Working in a factory I watched lots of supervisors and managers who shouted at people to get work done. I thought, there has to be another way to get people to work more productively. I did find people. But at the time (the early to mid-80s) they were very much in the minority. I was clear, I wanted to be more like the minority. I wanted to find a way to work with people, to bring out the best in them. Not shout at and humiliate them.

---

[47] Waitley, *The Psychology of Winning*, 1979.

Finding great people to help you is your biggest mission

If you take one piece of advice from this book, it's to find people who are passionate about what you want to do and who are working to become better version of themselves. These people are potential role models and gold dust for you. In reality, unless we are growing mentally and challenging ourselves, we are suffering a slow boring decline towards mental apathy and who wants that? Networking to find role models is a great skill that doesn't come naturally to everyone. But once you have found an approach you're comfortable with you will be unstoppable.

Your group of new people do not have to stutter. They should share your passion for self-improvement and have the skills or expertise that you want to master. Your aim is to find people who will help you achieve your goals. People will surprise you. Nine times out of 10, if you ask, they will help you.

Can you find more than five?

Jim Rohn, American entrepreneur, author and motivational speaker, says, 'You become the average of the five people you spend the most time with.'[48] He might be right! I know that if you surround yourself with people who have low ambition, low energy, the observers of life, it will harder for you to raise your head up. Go and find hungry, determined and passionate people. But don't stop at five. Your goal is to create a powerful network of people who inspire you to be better. And who you can learn from. You may get stick from your old crowd. But remember, they're happy where they are. You don't have to be!

---

[48] Ashley-Roberts, C., 'Are you ready to take your leadership to the next level?', 2020.

Your story exercise – find brilliant people to help you achieve your life goals

Brainstorm in your Success Workbook all the potential people you know who could help you achieve your goals. Or if you don't know people who can directly help you, do you know someone who does? Ask them to introduce you. Don't give up if that doesn't work. Do a review on the internet, who else could help you? Decide on your first action step to contact someone. And do it. Build your network of inspirational people to help you create the life you want. Be brave, this is your life we're talking about!

Summary of Step 5 – How do you get what you want?

The five objectives of Step 5 were:

1. Learning to use the Success Action Process to solve any problem
2. Understand your success is down to your mental metal
3. Make time to achieve your goals and own the first hour of the day
4. Write down what you are doing and take time to reflect and learn
5. Find role models you can learn from and who will help you

Part 3

Conclusion

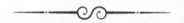

A stuttering revolution

We have covered a lot of ground together. I hope you have made significant progress in the creation and belief that you can have the life you really want, despite having a stutter. We have enough role models to know that we don't have to be fluent to be successful. I hope you have found the exercises useful and they have helped you to reflect on your story so far. More importantly, I hope that you have discovered a path to the next brilliant and exciting chapter of your life. I want to inspire people who stutter to take control of their lives using the five-step process, to take off their shackles and take action. That's why I want a stuttering revolution. And to ask you to join me in the fight to be heard for all that we really are.

I never needed fixing. I just needed someone to believe in me. In the end I had to find a way to believe in myself. It just took me a lot longer than I ever thought it would. I will share that defining moment with you shortly. It was an unexpected moment in work. I had a life-changing thought. A thought that changed my life. A revelation that completely changed the way I thought about me and my stutter.

I never needed fixing

From the moment my primary school teacher told me I had a stutter and it was psychological, I believed there was something wrong with me. And I needed fixing. This belief was reinforced by my parents taking me on a seven-year journey of medical treatments, trying to find a cure to fix their son and his stutter. No one ever stopped to think, ask or assume that I was OK. That I just happened to speak differently than other kids.

Research has established that stuttering is not our fault. And it's not a psychological problem that needs to be fixed. For two out of three people who stutter it's hereditary and therefore has a neurological basis. It's hard wiring in the brain. The blood is not getting to the places it needs to get to. Why is this important? If I had known about this research when I was younger, I wouldn't have thought there was something psychologically wrong with me. Which may have changed the way in which I was treated by the medical profession and by those around me. It might have also taken some pressure off my parents. And me. Who knows!

You and I may never be fluent. And that's OK; we don't need to be. As we have discussed throughout the book, it's time to focus on what you're good at and what you want from your life. What have you got to lose? I once saw a magazine advertisement for the American Stuttering Foundation which summed it up: there are many effective ways to improve stuttering – but doing nothing is not one of them. As you know, I'm suggesting that a stuttering revolution is to focus on the best of you!

If only society knew

Jo Biden, President of the United States, controversially said that stuttering 'is the only handicap people still laugh about'.[49] If there was wide-spread understanding that stuttering was not a psychological deficiency, then maybe the stigma attached to stuttering would stop. We wouldn't get laughed at, mocked, thought we are less intelligent

---

[49] Schwab, 'Joe Biden calls stuttering the "only handicap people still laugh about"', 2020.

or lazy, drunk or somehow inferior to other people. Global research tells us people who stutter are less likely to apply and be successful in getting a job, more likely to take jobs below our capability and less likely to be promoted than those who don't stutter. The potential, often unintended, discrimination can prevent organizations from finding and enabling much-needed talent. Us! We also know from the research that some people who stutter hold themselves back from the workplace or hide their stuttering for fear of failure, humiliation or ridicule. I know I've been humiliated and embarrassed on countless occasions because of the way I speak. Or, more accurately, because of the way I don't speak. You may have also had the same experience. I would encourage you to make a stand for you. You stutter. So what!! Build your confidence through the exercises in the book and don't let others affect your progress.

That's why I want a stuttering revolution.

There are an estimated 70 million adults of working age who stutter globally.[50] That's why I want a revolution in thinking. A step-by-step approach that 70 million people can do something to help themselves. To start to believe there could be a different way rather than focusing on the way we speak. Instead, to look at what we can do. To discover the life we dream about, to find a job we will love to do, and be successful in, to understand what we're already good at and develop our talents, skills and expertise into a superpower. If you really want to make a change in your life you can. No one is coming to rescue you. It's down to you to decide and take action. You can be who you want to be. You now have the tools. You'll find plenty of decent people in society who are kind, helpful and supportive. F-F-F-F-F-F-F-F-F-F-F-F-F-F-Forget the rest (a little stuttering joke there for you!).

---

[50] DoSomething.org, '11 facts about stuttering', n.d.

The world is full of stuttering role models

We can see in our daily lives the proof that I'm right to focus on what we do well rather than the way we speak. There are famous people in all walks of life who stutter, or who have stuttered in their past. Emily Blunt, Elon Musk, Ed Sheeran, Samuel L. Jackson, Darren Sproles, Noel Gallagher, Nicole Kidman, John Hendrickson and Tiger Woods, to name a few. All defying and proving many of the stigmas we face to be wrong. But there are also successful people who stutter, who may not be famous, in every walk of life. Politicians, speech therapists, doctors, vets, mathematicians, engineers, journalists, influencers, accountants, sales reps, retail assistants. If you name a trade or profession, someone who stutters is doing it. Today.

The first step is deciding

I took a decision when I was 17 years of age to stop all the medical treatment trying to fix me and my stutter. I decided I didn't want to be defined by the way I spoke. I also knew I wanted more from my life. This decision started me on a tough but insightful journey. I've had to stand up for myself, fight the doubting voices in my head and push myself to become more than my stutter. I now want to take all my learning and help others become whatever they want to be in life. People like you.

This is a story about your revolution

I know you've picked up this book because you want to help yourself. You want to take charge of your destiny. You know there is more of you to give the world. You know that stuttering is part of you, not all of you. I love the (anecdotal) quote from Abraham Lincoln who fought for another type of revolution. 'I abolished slavery and brought a nation together, and I was a stutterer.' The way he spoke didn't hold

Abe back! Are you still thinking about why or if you should try a different approach?

The five-step process will help you become so much more than your stutter

I've shared some of the stories of my journey to encourage you to share yours. Our journeys are like us. Unique. They shape who we become. After working around the world for over 20 years creating strategies to bring out the best in people, and being a lifelong stutterer, I wanted to create a practical process to help you on your journey to whatever is next for you.

The five steps are practical and contain exercises that I know work. Hopefully the five-step process has helped you to:

- Get to the truth of why you want to become more than your stutter, your desire
- Clarify what you really want out of your life, your ambition
- Discover the work you love to do, and what you need to love that work, your passion
- Identify your strengths, a potential superpower and any gaps you may need to address
- Learn five new skills that turn your thoughts into your new life

Most of the exercises you will only need to do once and capture in your Success Workbook, to create your Success Script and Success Summary Sheet. Once you have achieved a substantial number of your goals you will revisit your Success Script. I found a quick review every 90 days to be useful and then a big review every two or three years. Changing your Success Script is a bit like wanting to move house. You need to think a lot. Plan a lot. Make the move. But then you're done for a few years while you do up your new house and get the benefit from the move. Get the benefit from your Success Script. Get most of the work done. Then move on.

A personal revelation

I want to share a personal story of an unexpected insight into my life and my relationship with my stutter. I hope the story will really help change your thinking and the way you view you and your stutter.

At 17 I knew that I wanted to be an inspirational speaker. From starting my first job, I looked for opportunities to speak in front of an audience, even though it filled me with dread. I had an inner voice that wanted to create speeches to inspire people. I also wanted to entertain people and be funny. It became a mark of my character that I would push myself when I was obviously struggling to speak. Nothing would stop me saying what I needed to say. As my confidence in work grew and I started to move closer to jobs that I loved to do, I found a real ability to connect with an audience. I got better at presentations. But that wasn't enough. I wanted to be known as someone who was renowned for giving great presentations and speeches.

In 2006, Bob Guinness, CEO of the newly formed Serco Science Executive team (I was the human resources director), decided to hold a conference for the top 300 leaders in a big hotel in Brighton. The purpose of the conference was to set out our ambitious goals and inspire our leadership team to grow and significantly improve the performance of the business. Each member of the executive team was tasked to create a presentation. I was given the leadership presentation on Day 2 of the conference, just before the CEO's closing remarks. I was surprised. The leadership presentation was the finale of the conference and normally used to inspire, motivate and energize the leaders before they returned to their day jobs. I felt excited by the opportunity. But it also felt like a big responsibility. The Science Executive team were the best team I had ever worked with. They were super bright, talented and just great people. I didn't want to let them down. Never mind the 300 people in the audience. I just needed to get it right.

Focus on what I was passionate about

I immediately got stuck on what to say. I had too many ideas. I was muddled. I went to see Clare Sadler, an executive coach who I'd worked with for a number of years. After talking through a few ideas, she asked me to remember why I was a leader. Why was I passionate about doing the job I did? Why was I driven to be the best leader I could be? I knew the answers to those questions. I felt energized and inspired. I had the idea for my presentation.

I decided I really wanted to connect with the audience and ask the leaders what Clare had asked me. Why are you a leader? I wanted to help them remember where those feelings came from. And ask them how they would use those feelings to connect with who they were today and the goals and challenges they faced ahead of them?

Selfishly, I also wanted to make my presentation different. A bit quirky. Not your normal corporate presentation with PowerPoint slides and graphs. I wanted something people would remember for years to come. I also wanted to inspire myself.

Why is Saucepan Man in your presentation?

I decided to take a risk. I based the first part of my presentation on a book from my childhood, *The Magic Faraway Tree* by Enid Blyton. I planned to ask the audience about the books they had read when they were children. I would ask them to remember the heroes, the explorers and the adventurers that had inspired them. I wanted them to remember the first time they had ever felt a stirring, a feeling of wanting to lead others. The speech was 20 minutes long and also included short stories of real-life heroes from all walks of life who were role models and would inspire us all. I would finish the presentation with a call to arms and challenge the top 300 leaders to live up to our values, and to be the best leaders they could be. To inspire and lead 12,000 to build the most successful business we could. And do it in the right way.

Pre-presentation stuttering jitters

The gorilla in the room. My stutter was top of my mind. I would present just before the CEO's closing remarks. The voices in my head were loud. *You have rehearsed for hours, you'll be fine. This is really important for Bob and the executive team. You know he thinks it's wacky?* (He did, but god bless him he still let me do it.) *What are a bunch of scientists and engineers going to think? It's weird. Right?* But there was another voice. The one that knew I was capable of something special. I just had to push myself and believe I would be OK.

As I walked on to the stage I saw 300 expectant and slightly puzzled faces. The conference audio team whispered the names of the audience through the speakers to sound like the rustling leaves of *The Enchanted Wood*. I had a wok in my left hand, a frying pan in my right hand and two pans tied with string hanging round my neck. (I was dressed how I imagined Saucepan Man would look.) And I began…

When it all comes together in that moment

When you love what you do, and you're doing what you love, there are moments when time stops still. I have read that tennis players at the top of their game can see the ball moving in slow motion. Great footballers seem to have more time on the ball. Authors write a book and don't know where the time went. I was half way into my speech and the audience appeared spellbound. I felt I had them in the palm of my hand. I could feel the changes of energy and emotion in the audience as I went through each part of my story. I felt like I was in slow motion.

The sudden realization caused me to pause for a millisecond. A very quick voice popped up, 'a block? No, I'm fine. Crack on.' I could feel my emotion and that of the audience building to a crescendo for the finale. The call to arms. A challenge to them all to inspire and lead 12,000 people to build the best business they could, always living to a set of shared values. I nailed it!

A standing ovation

I finished speaking. I paused. There was a strange moment of silence. *Yikes!*, I thought. It's not worked. Then the applause. A standing ovation. Hollers, whoops, cheers. This was a very traditional British, science nuclear and engineering-based audience. They don't normally do that. Many had tears in their eyes, including the executive team. I was just relieved it had worked.

In that moment of applause, I was lost deep in thought. My world seemed to be moving in slow motion. I remembered at 17 having a dream that one day I would inspire an audience from a stage. At 17, I knew I wanted to go somewhere. But I didn't know where I was going. At 17, I had days when I could barely speak. And here I was, giving the speech of my life. In that moment I knew my stutter was no longer holding me back. Maybe it never had?

But there was something else. A thought that seemed to come from nowhere. But a feeling I felt everywhere. I had a thought that changed my life. A life-changing thought. A revelation that blew my mind. I realized for the first time that the only thing that had ever held me back was me!

What does the revelation mean for you?

You can spend a lot of time and energy trying to become fluent. Or you can spend the same amount of time and energy focusing on what you want from your life. What you're passionate about. And develop yourself to become so much more than your stutter. Your stutter is part of you. Not all of you. Don't hide behind it. Believe with certainty. You are more. You are the only thing holding you back. Not your stutter.

You may still look for support to improve the way you communicate with others. We should all strive to be better communicators (people who stutter and those who don't). But do it with the confidence that improving the way you communicate with others, the way you speak, is part of you. Not all of you. This is why I want you to join me in the 'stuttering revolution'. Make a stand for you and the estimated 70 million other adults and god knows how many children who stutter around the world who have more to give!

Next, you'll be saying you've benefited from having a stutter

You're absolutely right, I am. I love the quote from David Seidler, who won an Oscar, BAFTA and so many more awards for his film, *The King's Speech*. 'If you can live through a childhood of stuttering, you can live through anything. And if you go into adulthood still stuttering, you can handle anything. You have been tempered by the fire.'[51] You and I know this is true!

I genuinely believe that my stutter has given me a lot to be thankful for. I just couldn't see it when I was younger. Because I have spent so much time on introspection, learning how to improve myself, watching and learning what does and doesn't work, I now have a huge appreciation and understanding of the following:

- My struggle with my stutter has made me resilient in many areas of my life
- Having to push myself to be heard and achieve my goals has made me determined

---

[51] Rossi, 'I am a man who stutters', 2014.

- Getting to know people beyond what they first say and how they say it
- How to laugh at myself and not take me, too seriously
- Using humour to put other people at ease with their discomfort of my stutter
- Being adaptable in my communication with others: if one way doesn't work, try another
- How to have personal steel and make a stand for me when I need it
- Working around the world to learn how to bring out the best in many people of many nationalities
- Disagreements are often misunderstandings of language and a different view of the world
- Fearless asking of questions without feeling stupid
- My passion to help and coach others, be it whatever they want to become
- Everyone has demons and voices in their head
- My fascination to focus on people's difference as a strength and not as a weapon to isolate
- The need of everyone to feel they are part of something that has purpose beyond them

There is so much more. As bizarre as it sounds, I'm grateful for my stutter and the struggles I have been through. I would not be the person I am today without my stutter. I have realized that I'm not really trying to become more than my stutter. I'm trying to become more. I want to learn and grow and push myself. I just happen to have a stutter. So what! In researching this book, I have become far more aware of the many, many fabulous people who have pushed through their stutter, and their struggles for a life they want to live. They have all realized having a better life was down to them. I admire them all immensely. I watch in awe those who have achieved their goals and ambitions. What do you think? Has your stutter benefited you in any way? I'm sure it has!

Don't fix your stutter, fix your life

I will end as I started, with Joe Biden, the president of the United States of America. I don't hold any political view. But I believe the quote from Joe Biden expresses the overall intent behind *A Stuttering Revolution*:

> If I could share one piece of advice for those of you who are struggling with a stutter, it would be this: when you commit yourself to a goal and when you persevere in the face of a struggle, you will discover new strengths, and skills, to help you overcome not only this challenge, but future life challenges as well. I promise you, you have nothing to be ashamed of, and you have every reason to be proud.[52]

As you have worked through the five-step process you have identified what you want to achieve in your life. You know the type of job you will love to do. You understand what you are good at and what you could develop into a superpower. Like Joe Biden says, you have committed to achieving all that you set out to achieve in your Success Script. We have called this desire, the determination to achieve our goals despite whatever is thrown at us.

Along the way you will encounter people who tell you that you cannot succeed. And that you will fail. There will be unforeseen challenges and moments of self-doubt. But you now have a set of tools and techniques that will help you overcome any obstacle that you will undoubtedly face. Including a network of brilliant people who you have selected to help you succeed on your journey. You now have a new set of skills that will build and develop your armoury to fight, to make a stand, to show the world that you are more than your stutter. Remember, your stutter is part of you. Not all of you!

---

[52] Stuttering Foundation, 'President Joe Biden', 2021.

Imagine how proud you will feel when you're achieving your goals! Imagine how proud your family and friends will feel when they see you becoming the you that you really want to be. The pride you will feel in the knowledge that you have not let your stutter limit or define you. You have worked to discover what you really want from you and your life. And that inner voice, that true version of you, is looking back at you in the mirror every day. You have become a better you.

So now you know. Your stutter is not stopping you. Over to you!

Appendices

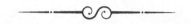

Success Summary Sheet

We will create a one page Summary Sheet of your Workbook				
One or two sentences that describe your overall ambitions and goals				
DESIRE	AMBITION		PASSION	
Fuel	Goals within 1 year	Goals within 3 years	Work You Love to Do	Loving the Work you Do
10				
9				
8				
7				
6	STRENGTHS			
5	Talent you have today	Gaps to close	Build Super Power	
4				
3	SUCCESS ROUTINES			
2	Daily Hour - time	Weekly Journal time and day	New Network Targets	
1				

Fig. 4 Your life plan. On a single page.

Organizations with contact details – support for people who stutter

During the writing of the book, I discovered a world of help that I hadn't known existed. I have looked at all the organizations listed below, and I know there is something which or someone who could help or support you on your journey within them.

STAMMA – The British Stammering Organisation
https://stamma.org

Michael Palin Centre for Stammering
https://michaelpalincentreforstammering.org

Stammering – UK National Health Service
www.nhs/conditions/stammering

The McGuire Programme – Beyond Stuttering
www.mcguireprogramme.com

American Institute for Stuttering
www.stutteringtreatment.org

The Stuttering Foundation
www.stutteringhelp.org

Further resources

A wide range of resources and help in support of the book can be found at the following websites:

https://astutteringrevolution.com (includes my TEDx talk, 'A Stuttering Revolution')

astutteringrevolution.co.uk

paulgaskin.co.uk

References

Anderson, B. M. (2022, May 16). '15 jobs you'll be recruiting for in 2030'. *LinkedIn Talent Blog.* www.linkedin.com/business/talent/blog/talent-strategy/jobs-you-will-be-recruiting-for-in-2030

Ashley-Roberts, C. (2020). 'Are you ready to take your leadership to the next level?'. *Your Time to Grow.* https://yourtimetogrow.com/ready-to-take-leadership-next-level/

Barnes, H. (2021, October 29). 'Einstein, visualization, and your career'. *Harrison Barnes.* www.harrisonbarnes.com/einstein-visualization-and-your-career

Berman, M. (2021, July 29). '10 desire quotes to help you build a burning desire for success'. *Programming Insider.* https://programminginsider.com/10-desire-quotes-to-help-you-build-a-burning-desire-for-success/

Bilyeu, L. (n.d.) 'When Tom asked my dad for his blessing, he said … no!' *Instagram.* www.instagram.com/p/B86Jl6EHWm5/?hl=en

Bilyeu, T. (2018, December 11). 'Become a savage & live on your own terms! | David Goggins'. *YouTube.* www.youtube.com/watch?v=dIM7E8e9JKY

Bose, S. D. (2022, September 8). 'When Jim Carrey wrote himself a $10 million cheque'. *Far Out Magazine.* https://faroutmagazine.co.uk/jim-carrey-wrote-himself-10-million-cheque/

Bridges, W., & Bridges, S. (2019). *Transitions: Making Sense of Life's Changes.* Da Capo Lifelong Books.

Brighton, T. (2010). *Patton, Montgomery, Rommel: Masters of War.* Three Rivers Press.

Buckingham, M., & Coffman, C. (2014). *First, Break All the Rules: What the World's Greatest Managers Do Differently.* Simon and Schuster.

Byers, T. (2022). 'The power of the mind through visualization'. *Swimming World News.* www.swimmingworldmagazine.com/news/the-power-of-the-mind-through-visualization/

Carnegie, D. (1991). *How to Win Friends and Influence People.* Vermillion.

Charvet, S. R. (1997). *Words That Change Minds.* Kendall/Hunt.

Chopra, D. (1996). *The Seven Spiritual Laws of Success, A Practical Guide to the Fulfilment of your Dreams.* Bantam Press.

Clifford, C. (2020, November 20). 'Apple CEO Tim Cook: "If you love what you do, you will never work a day in your life" is "total crock"'. *CNBC.* www.cnbc.com/2019/05/18/apple-ceo-tim-cook-if-you-love-what-you-do-you-will-never-work-a-day-in-your-life-is-total-crock.html

Clifton, B. J. (2023, January 16). 'The world's broken workplace'. *Gallup.* https://news.gallup.com/opinion/chairman/212045/world-broken-workplace.aspx

Coelho, P. (2011). *The Fifth Mountain.* HarperCollins UK.

Colan, L. (2020, February 6). 'A lesson from Roy A. Disney on making values-based decisions'. *Inc.com.* www.inc.com/lee-colan/a-lesson-from-roy-a-disney-on-making-values-based-decisions.html

Covey, R. S. (1994). *The Seven Habits of Highly Effective People, Powerful Lessons in Personal Change.* Simon & Schuster.

Dance, A. (2020, September 4). 'What neuroscientists are discovering about stuttering'. *Smithsonian Magazine*. www.smithsonianmag.com/science-nature/what-neuroscientists-are-discovering-about-stuttering-180975730/#:~:text=These%20findings%20hint%20that%20stuttering,be%20coordinated%20at%20lightning%20speed

Descartes, R., & Cress, D. A. (1998). *Discourse on Method (Third Edition)*. Hackett Publishing.

DoSomething.org. (n.d.). '11 facts about stuttering'. www.dosomething.org/us/facts/11-facts-about-stuttering

Drake, A. (2022). 'VALLEY tries it: Robin Sharma's 20/20/20 method of the 5 a.m. club'. *VALLEY Magazine*. www.valleymagazinepsu.com/valley-tries-it-robin-sharmas-20-20-20-method-of-the-5-a-m-club/

Einstein, A., & Shaw, G. B. (2012). *Einstein on Cosmic Religion and Other Opinions and Aphorisms*. Courier Corporation.

Eker, T. H. (2005). *Secrets of the Millionaire Mind*. Harper Business.

Fisher, J. F. (2019, December 27). 'How to get a job often comes down to one elite personal asset, and many people still don't realize it'. *CNBC Work*. www.cnbc.com/2019/12/27/how-to-get-a-job-often-comes-down-to-one-elite-personal-asset.html

Foster, J. (2013, May 11). 'Whether you think you can ... or whether you think you can't ... you're right!' *Wall Street Insanity*. https://wallstreetinsanity.com/whether-you-think-you-can-or-whether-you-think-you-cant-youre-right/

Gates, G. (n.d.). 'Gareth Gates – stop my stutter'. *BBC Three*. www.bbc.co.uk/blogs/bbcthree/2012/02/gareth-gates-stop-my-stutter.shtml

George, B. and Sims, P. (2007). *True North, Discover your Authentic Leadership*, Jossey-Bass.

Goggins, D. (n.d.). www.facebook.com/iamdavidgoggins/photos/a.51
8497645028266/548765868668110/?type=3

Goggins, D. (2020). *Can't Hurt Me: Master Your Mind and Defy the
Odds – Clean Edition*. Lioncrest Publishing.

Hamre, E. (2021, December 16). 'Tom Bilyeu's most inspirational
advice on how to achieve greatness'. *Medium.* https://medium.com/
skilluped/tom-bilyeus-most-inspirational-advice-on-how-to-achieve-
greatness-36e9a02155b7

Helmstetter, S. (1990). *What to Say When You Talk to Your Self.* Simon
and Schuster.

Hill, E. (2022, July 1). 'Stuttering "American Idol" contestant steals the
spotlight'. *Parade.* https://parade.com/131649/erinhill/18-american-
idol-stuttering-contestant

Hill, N. (2004). *Think and Grow Rich*. Random House.

I'Anson, J. (2012, November 23). 'How to find unadvertised jobs'. *The
Guardian*, Careers Blog. www.theguardian.com/careers/careers-blog/
how-to-find-unadvertised-jobs

Jay-Z (2010). *Decoded*. Random House.

Jeffers, S. (2007). *Feel The Fear And Do It Anyway: How to Turn Your
Fear and Indecision into Confidence and Action*. Edbury Publishing.

Klein, J., & Hood, S. (2004). 'The impact of stuttering on employment
opportunities and job performance'. *Journal of Fluency Disorders*,
29(4), 255–273. https://doi.org/10.1016/j.jfludis.2004.08.001

Krasuski, J. (2019, July 10). 'Regret avoidance – LifeBrief psychiatry
blog'. *LifeBrief.* www.lifebrief.com/regret-avoidance/

Kushel, G. (1985). *The 4%: How to Be One of the 4% Who Enjoy Total Success in Both Their Personal and Work Lives - the Fully Effective Executives.* Pan Macmillan.

Lally, P., van Jaarsveld, C. H. M., Potts, H. W. W., & Wardle, J. (2010). 'How are habits formed: modelling habit formation in the real world'. *European Journal of Social Psychology,* 40, 998–1009. https://doi.org/10.1002/ejsp.674

Lee, A. (2016, June 7). 'Bruce Willis gets emotional in speech on stuttering: "Never let anyone make you feel like an outcast"'. *The Hollywood Reporter.* www.hollywoodreporter.com/news/general-news/bruce-willis-stuttering-never-let-900434/

Maltz, M. (2022). *Psycho-Cybernetics (Updated and Expanded).* Souvenir Press.

McConaughey, M. (2020). *Greenlights.* Headline.

Obama, M. (2018). *Becoming.* Crown.

Ofcom (2020). 'Online nation, 2020 report'. www.ofcom.org.uk/__data/assets/pdf_file/0027/196407/online-nation-2020-report.pdf

Ofcom (2022, February 21). 'Children and parents: media use and attitudes report 2020/21'. www.ofcom.org.uk/research-and-data/media-literacy-research/childrens/children-and-parents-media-use-and-attitudes-report-2021

Peterson, J. B. (n.d.). www.facebook.com/drjordanpeterson/photos/a.540348442695962/2655421477855304/?type=3

Rivers, C. (2022, January 21). 'Successful people use visualization'. *EnVision.* https://envision.app/2019/08/22/successful-people-use-visualization-techniques/

Robbins, A. (1986). *Unlimited Power.* Ballantine Books.

Robbins, M. [@melrobbins] (2017, November 29). 'Don't miss out on your life because you're too busy scrolling through someone else's'. *Twitter*. Retrieved June 29, 2023, from https://twitter.com/melrobbins/status/935706886560800773?lang=en-GB

Robbins, T. (1992). *Awaken the Giant Within: How to Take Immediate Control of Your Mental, Emotional, Physical and Financial Destiny!* Simon & Schuster.

Rossi, D. (2014). 'I am a man who stutters'. *The Good Men Project*. https://goodmenproject.com/featured-content/cc-i-am-a-man-who-stutters/

Schwab, N. (2020, February 6). 'Joe Biden calls stuttering the "only handicap people still laugh about"'. *Mail Online*. www.dailymail.co.uk/news/article-7972021/Joe-Biden-calls-stuttering-handicap-people-laugh-about.html

Shahbaz, A. (2020, November 12). 'What Joe Biden's speech disorder means for young Americans with disabilities'. *Forbes*. www.forbes.com/sites/alishahbaz/2020/11/12/what-joe-bidens-speech-disorder-means-for-young-americans-with-disabilities

Sharma, R. S. (2021). *The Monk Who Sold His Ferrari: Special 25th Anniversary Edition*. HarperCollins.

Sheehan, J. G. (1970). *Stuttering: Research and Therapy*. Harper & Row.

Smulders, D. (2022). '100 lessons from Tony Robbins' "Unleash the Power Within 2018"'. *WUA*. https://wua.cx/klaas-kroezen-my-top-100-lessons-after-going-with-the-team-to-tony-robbins-in-london/

Stamurai (2021, December 15). 'Do you know about Ed Sheeran's stuttering journey?' *Medium*. https://stamuraiapp.medium.com/do-you-know-about-ed-sheerans-stuttering-journey-40740d8589e5

Stanford News (2005, 12 June). '"You've got to find what you love," Jobs says'. https://news.stanford.edu/2005/06/12/youve-got-find-love-jobs-says/

Stuttering Foundation: A Nonprofit Organization Helping Those Who Stutter (2015, October 26). 'Actor Sam Neill talks about stuttering'. www.stutteringhelp.org/content/actor-sam-neill-talks-about-stuttering

Stuttering Foundation: A Nonprofit Organization Helping Those Who Stutter (2021, January 12). 'Darren Sproles'. www.stutteringhelp.org/famous-people/darren-sproles

Stuttering Foundation: A Nonprofit Organization Helping Those Who Stutter (2021, March 8). 'President Joe Biden'. www.stutteringhelp.org/content/president-joe-biden

Suffolk Center for Speech (n.d.) 'Darren Sproles – a football player who stutters'. www.lispeech.com/darren-sproles-a-football-player-who-stutters/

Udland, M. (2015, November 11). 'Warren Buffett thinks working just to beef up your résumé is like "saving up sex for your old age"' *Insider*, www.businessinsider.com/warren-buffett-on-resume-building-2015-11?r=US&IR=T

Van Eerd, R., & Guo, J. (2020, January 17). 'Jobs will be very different in 10 years. Here's how to prepare'. *World Economic Forum – Future of Work*. www.weforum.org/agenda/2020/01/future-of-work/

Waitley, D. (1979). *The Psychology of Winning*. Berkley Books. https://ci.nii.ac.jp/ncid/BA36994372

Wilcox, A. (2021, December 15). 'The law of attraction will never be enough'. *Medium*. https://medium.com/@aliciawilcox/the-law-of-attraction-will-never-be-enough-8e584e851ec8

INDEX

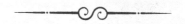

A quick word from Practical Inspiration Publishing...

We hope you found this book both practical and inspiring – that's what we aim for with every book we publish.

We publish titles on topics ranging from leadership, entrepreneurship, HR and marketing to self-development and wellbeing.

Find details of all our books at: www.practicalinspiration.com

 Did you know...

We can offer discounts on bulk sales of all our titles – ideal if you want to use them for training purposes, corporate giveaways or simply because you feel these ideas deserve to be shared with your network.

We can even produce bespoke versions of our books, for example with your organization's logo and/or a tailored foreword.

To discuss further, contact us on info@practicalinspiration.com.

 Got an idea for a business book?

We may be able to help. Find out more about publishing in partnership with us at: bit.ly/PIpublishing.

Follow us on social media...

 @PIPTalking

 @pip_talking

 @practicalinspiration

 @piptalking

 Practical Inspiration Publishing

Printed in the USA
CPSIA information can be obtained
at www.ICGtesting.com
JSHW012022130524
63048JS00007B/370